Dementia:
What You Need to Know

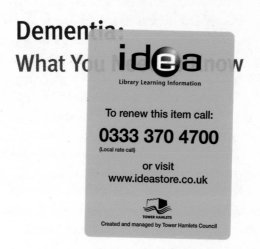

June Andrews is Professor Emeritus in Dementia Studies at the University of Stirling in Scotland. She has worked in hospitals, nursing organisations and government and currently sits on the boards of health and social care organisations and businesses. June is the co-author of *10 Helpful Hints for Carers*, on helping care for those with dementia. In 2014 she was awarded a fellowship by the Royal College of Nursing and in 2016 was awarded an OBE in the Queen's 90th Birthday Honours list for services to people with dementia. She is author of *Dementia: the One-Stop Guide*.

Dementia:
What You Need to Know

*Practical advice for families, professionals and people
living with dementia and Alzheimer's disease around
the world*

Professor June Andrews

PROFILE BOOKS

The advice provi[...]
checked by the au[...]
regarded as a sub[...]
additional inform[...]
that have changed[...]

First published in 2016 by
PROFILE BOOKS LTD
3 Holford Yard
Bevin Way
London
WC1X 9HD
www.profilebooks.com

Designed and typeset by sue@lambledesign.demon.co.uk
Printed and bound by CPI Group (UK) Ltd, Croydon, CR0 4YY

ISBN 978 1 78125 670 1
eISBN 978 1 84765 991 0

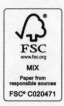

FSC
www.fsc.org
MIX
Paper from
responsible sources
FSC® C020471

Contents

To the memory of Frank Hitchman (1942–2016).
A fine gentleman, patron of the arts and Secretary to the
Dementia Services Development Trust.

Foreword

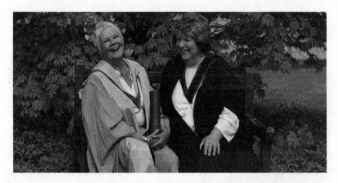

Dame Judi Dench with Professor June Andrews, Iris Murdoch
Centre, July 2013

Dear reader

I knew nothing really of dementia before working on
the film biography of Iris Murdoch. I was delighted
to have played the part of Iris and learned a great deal
about this condition from others working on the project
who had direct experience of Alzheimer's disease. I'm
very, very pleased that if the film did anything, it put
this illness into the spotlight for perhaps the first time.
In the years since I undertook this role, I have watched
the dementia work of the Iris Murdoch Centre at the

University of Stirling and become an ambassador for those who help people with Alzheimer's disease, doing what I can to support them in raising awareness.

This book became an instant best seller in the UK because it is so clear and practical and I commend this international edition to you.

It was very daunting playing the role of a woman with dementia for a film, but it must be so much harder to live through the experience. I hope this book will help families and friends of people with dementia all over the world, and be a support to those professionals who work to improve their difficult journey.

With love and all good wishes

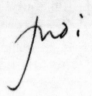

Introduction

This book is about dementia and what happens when someone is affected by it. The word 'dementia' is used to describe the collection of warning signs that show up when your brain stops working as well as it used to. It is defined as dementia only if these signs continue to get worse, with a permanent deterioration over time. If you know about dementia you will be better able to look after yourself or someone in your family who is affected by it.

Interest in dementia in the media has never been so great. Movies have been made about famous people who had dementia. *Iris*, starring Dame Judi Dench, tells the true story of the English novelist Iris Murdoch from her brilliant youth to her last days in a care home. *The Iron Lady* is a moving film which explores the former UK Prime Minister Margaret Thatcher's life through fragments of history that represent her disintegrating thinking and recollection clouded by dementia (and some rather impressive hallucinations). Movies also explore ethical issues. *Away from Her*, *Still Alice* and *The Savages* describe the dilemmas and family dynamics of caring. Although there is still stigma, this public airing means that people are more open about dementia and allow themselves to think about it more than they did in the past. This is all good.

Public figures affected by dementia in their families are recruited as champions by dementia charities and encouraged to talk publicly about dementia and share their stories with other people. Often when I get into a cab and the driver asks me what I do, I hear a personal story about how dementia has affected their family. Once upon a time it was a shameful secret.

Nevertheless, it is almost impossible to get sensible advice about dementia. We are faced with waves of publicity on the subject as newspapers print misleading headlines implying that there will be miracle cures available almost immediately. Families affected by dementia live in fear of losing their entire life's savings in care home fees. Television commercials encourage us to be positive about dementia while at the same time celebrities and thought leaders say that they'd rather have cancer, or that they believe they'd have a duty to kill themselves if they had dementia. Investigative reporters make TV shows out of the misery of vulnerable people who have been on the receiving end of bad care. Scandalous nursing-home stories ruin our confidence that there might be a place anywhere in which residents, even if they deteriorate, have the benefit of comfort and good cheer. The often-reported heartbreaking treatment of patients with dementia in hospital makes us afraid for ourselves and our older relatives.

In the middle of all this, thousands of people every year get the shocking news that someone in their family has dementia. For many of them their experience unfolds as if no one has ever travelled this path before. They are in uncharted territory, often surrounded by professionals, family and friends who don't know a huge amount about the condition. For many people it is hard to know where to turn for sensible advice.

How do I know this? In 2011, with Professor Allan House, a liaison psychiatrist, I wrote a book in plain language called *10 Helpful Hints for Carers* based on the existing research. Our printers' proof copies kept being 'borrowed' by doctors, who did not return them. When it was published, families read it avidly. In the following years nearly 65,000 copies had been sold, or exchanged for donations for the Dementia Services Development Trust, the charity that supported us. Families said, 'Why did no one ever tell us these things before?' Professionals and volunteers took more and more copies, to give to patients, to families and to fellow workers who had never been taught about dementia in their training. At last there was some sensible and practical advice for anyone trying to make things better for people with dementia. But it was not enough. A second book *Dementia – the One-Stop Guide* was written for families in the UK. Readers welcomed the practical information and advice about how to cope with the dementia journey the best way possible but those outside the UK were frustrated that it was too specific to that single healthcare system. Now this volume has been written which will hopefully give some help to families anywhere in the world.

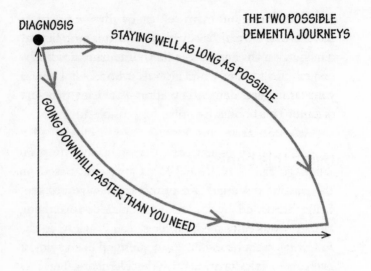

DIAGNOSIS

STAYING WELL AS LONG AS POSSIBLE

THE TWO POSSIBLE
DEMENTIA JOURNEYS

GOING DOWNHILL FASTER THAN YOU NEED

Everyone has a unique experience, but in general there are two possible routes with dementia. On one track you stay as well as possible for as long as possible, living life the way you want to. On the other, you go downhill faster than you need to, for reasons that are often avoidable. Everyone would like to avoid unnecessary trouble and expense, and to delay some of the difficult situations that might arise. Sensible, practical advice on how to do this is in short supply. People aren't told about the remarkable services and equipment that are readily available or the simple changes to their lifestyle which can be so radical that they prevent the need to go into a care home.

Dementia: What You Need to Know provides information about what will make a difference in the lives of people with dementia, their carers and caregivers. It is practical and compact, and builds on the *One-Stop*

Guide. In setting out to write this, I've drawn on information that is freely available if you've got a clinical qualification that prepares you to understand it and a few months to research it. However, when someone in your family gets dementia you may not have that sort of time. This book is for you.

Using this book

The idea of this guide is to provide as much information as possible in a portable form. Some people have read previous editions like a novel, from start to finish, and they say they found it really useful, but they noted that some advice is repeated. There's a reason for that. Some carers and people with dementia are so busy, they might dip into the book, and so if something is worth saying against more than one topic, it is mentioned under each, sometimes with a cross reference to the last time it was described, in case you are only reading one chapter at any time.

A note for health and social care professionals and care workers – some have thought of this as a book for families and carers, rather than professionals. This book is absolutely for you as well. You can either give it to your patient or client, or you can read it yourself and use it as a script for useful things you can tell them in your clinical encounter, or when you are advising them while working alongside them at home.

My aim is to base what I say on research. You won't find many footnotes or references here, but I am happy to take questions if you think that there is research that contradicts what the book says. Time passes and new things are found through time. So though I am light on academic language and style, this book is fundamentally focused on what is practical, makes a difference and is based on evidence.

Dementia: What You Need to Know has a lot of the same information as *Dementia – the One-Stop Guide* but where possible it has been updated with any new research since that book was written, and enriched by comments from readers who have given feedback and the generosity of professional colleagues. Because it covers what happens in a number of states, regions and countries, I've given a lot of references to websites and other sources of information. The fragmentation of care systems makes work for carers, but there are organisations listed here that can help.

chapter 1

What is dementia?

People use the term 'dementia' to mean a number of things. This chapter will give you a basic understanding of the commonest types of dementia and why it is useful to know the difference between them for practical reasons. Dementia is much more than just a memory problem. You might find that some of the professionals you meet are misinformed about it, so the more you know the better.

A range of diseases can cause the changes in the brain that give rise to dementia symptoms. There are probably more than a hundred of these diseases, but three or four of them are very common. The commonest is Alzheimer's disease. Up until recently student doctors and nurses were told little if anything about dementia. And if they were told anything, it was sometimes wrong. They were told not to worry about what underlying ailment was causing the patient to have the dementia signs and symptoms. This way of thinking was known by real experts to be wrong long before it was ever corrected in the education of the professionals. It was lazy thinking, which was inexcusable, even though there was not enough research on the subject to provide a huge amount of advice.

What did they used to say in the past? In my own experience I've heard all of these misleading statements … and there are more:

- It's just a memory problem.
- We shouldn't worry patients about this because we can't be sure of the diagnosis.
- Because you can't really tell for sure what disease is causing the problem until the autopsy, there's little point in diagnosing.
- There is no reason to raise the question of an underlying disease with the patient or their family because there is nothing that can be done.
- The treatment is the same no matter what the cause, so even the doctors and nurses don't need to distinguish between the possible causes of dementia.
- It's part of normal ageing – you expect and accept these symptoms in old people.
- It's a wasting disease – you can expect them to lose weight and die quite quickly.

In the course of this chapter I'll show that these assertions were wrong, but you need to be aware that this is what was taught to very many of the doctors, nurses, social workers and other professionals you might meet. You'll end up knowing more than they do. But you have to work with these people, so how you handle that difference in your level of knowledge can be tricky. The situation is getting better with all the recent public interest in dementia, but research shows that even if the professionals who are now working in the system received any dementia education in their undergraduate or pre-registration training, it was more likely to be about the anatomy and physiology of the declining brain tissue than about answers to practical questions: like what you should do if the person starts getting lost in the night. I hesitate to say that it was useless, but certainly the education has not been good enough from the point of view of caregivers or people with dementia who come looking for help. Most of the people with dementia seen by students in the past were in hospital and largely unable to do even the most basic tasks, and often they were behaving in very disturbing ways. That's how medical people viewed dementia – they expected dramatic and painful debilitation and chaos. They never realised that the majority of people with dementia were living quietly at home.

Things are a bit better now. There is a lot of publicity and more education. In some countries all the people who have been formally diagnosed with dementia are on a register. In the UK they are listed on a register at their family doctor's office, so that they can be considered for help, treatment and support. (At least they should be … in some cases the clinic doing the diagnosis fails to communicate it to the family doctor. Poor communication is an issue to be discussed later in the book.) In Scotland, caregivers are given a right to support through this listing. The health departments in the UK provide an incentive to family doctors by giving them an extra payment for putting people on the register. So that's good. What's more, many people are getting their diagnosis (*if* they get a diagnosis) at earlier stages of the condition, when they still have a lot of independence and can enjoy life, exercising their capacity to make decisions and have fun. That early diagnosis also means that they have more potential benefit from the limited range of medication that is available and can plan their future better.

In most other countries, there is no register, so the doctors and others in the field don't really know how much unmet need there is in the system. When they are planning a service, it would be much more useful to have some idea of what is going to be needed. If they are measuring how good their service is, they should have some idea at least of whether they are identifying the people who have the problem and offering them the right help.

Not everyone thinks that registers are a good idea, and in some countries the health system is so fragmented, that setting one up is tough. It's regarded as a good way of measuring if those who need care are likely to be getting it, but concerns about privacy and stigma, and resistance from doctors to the idea that diagnosis is useful are still issues of concern. Sweden has a register that is highly respected.

In countries with high incomes, the increase in the number of people with dementia has not been as fast as in the low-to-medium income countries. In Argentina, for example, the population has aged faster than anticipated. So the National Health Department is setting up a register called the RDeCAr, to track people with cognitive problems. In India it has been estimated that nine out of ten people with dementia have not been diagnosed even though India is experiencing a surge in numbers who are affected. In the USA people from minority ethnic populations who have dementia are referred to services later than white Americans. That means they may have more problems when they eventually see the services and they might even be in crisis. Later in this book it will be demonstrated that even though we don't like to think about it, the sooner you get to grips with this problem and see a doctor, the better it is for you and your family.

Everywhere in the world when you ask the question 'Is this dementia?' you are still dependent on a doctor to put a name to the troubling symptoms that have beset you or your loved one. If the family doctor remembers his or her training and it was as bad as mine was, they may not feel confident enough to make a diagnosis, and might still believe there is no point in trying. This means that you might have to push for that diagnosis. In some countries you are more likely to be referred to a neurologist, and in others, the work is done by specialist psychiatrists who might take advice from neurology. Variation is a problem. Even where the four health care systems of four countries are really similar (Scotland, England, Northern Ireland, Wales), there is huge difference. At the time of the first edition of this book, in Scotland and Northern Ireland two-thirds to three-quarters of people with dementia symptoms will have been formally diagnosed. In some parts of England as few as 20 per cent of people with dementia symptoms got their diagnosis. In total on average across all of England it was less than half and the same was true in France. In other countries without registers it might be hard to say how the numbers are going.

Particularly when they are older or if someone in their family has had dementia, people worry about whether they themselves are getting dementia. It's all over the news, and in surveys lots of people say they'd rather have cancer, so it is clearly terrifying. Sometimes people who think they have it try to hide it. Couples collude with each other, pretending that everything is all right when it isn't. Children worry about their parents and may be fearful of raising the subject. Friends don't like to mention it in case they cause offence. That's understandable, but there is no justification for any doctor to still actively avoid addressing the issue, though some clearly do.

What can you – as families and patients – do, given all the rules about patient confidentiality, if you have difficulty getting your doctor to take your concerns seriously? The first step is to find out for yourself as much as you can about dementia and the associated problems. That will give you power.

Things that look like dementia but aren't

Mild cognitive impairment

There is a condition called *mild cognitive impairment* (MCI), which many of us will get if we are lucky enough to grow old. Because some people who get dementia start with MCI it can be very worrying to have it. But cheer up! Lots of studies indicate that the majority of individuals with this memory loss never progress to having full-blown dementia, and MCI itself can sometimes be reversed or at least remain stable. You need to know what to do about MCI and how not to worry, but you also need to be sure to see a doctor if you really think it is progressing to become dementia.

If you have MCI, you may have minor difficulties with memory and attention, and some language issues. It is like being mentally tired all the time. In fact it can be brought on by stress and fatigue, or another illness, but unlike dementia it is potentially reversible and not necessarily progressive.

People with MCI have problems that are less extreme than people with dementia. At least 5 per cent of older people have MCI, depending on how you define it. It would be really useful if you could tell which of those are going to go on to develop dementia, but till now there has been no real way of knowing, so that means there is a limit to what doctors can do. There is some evidence that brain exercises might help, and all the things that you will read about later in this book that help reduce dementia symptoms are probably sensible to consider as a precaution in MCI.

Delirium

Another condition, called *delirium*, is a fluctuating temporary confusion that often happens to older people when they are ill because of something else, such as a urine infection, or too many medicines, or a chest infection. Delirium can be dangerous if it is not treated and people die as a result. Sometimes it is an early sign that the person is likely to get dementia in years to come, so if you've had it your doctor needs to be told. If delirium occurs in hospital, it may not get treated because staff see the older person in bed being 'confused' and don't think there is anything abnormal with that. It is vital that they not only treat it, but make sure that people understand its significance, as it can be an indication of vulnerability to dementia in future. As is made clear in Chapter 12, you need to make sure medical and nursing staff know if the level of confusion displayed at any time is a radical change and a deterioration from how the person usually is and you need to persuade the doctors and nurses to treat the cause.

Depression

In addition, if an older person gets depression, that may look a lot like dementia. Fortunately, depression can be treated and reversed. It is tragic if the health care staff wrongly assume that it is dementia and that therefore nothing can be done (because they are then wrong on two counts, as both dementia and depression can be helped). Family care givers need to be on their toes to make sure that unintended harm does not occur either because some doctors don't diagnose delirium or depression or dementia, or because they try but their diagnosis is wrong.

What are the symptoms of dementia?

The key symptoms of dementia include difficulty in:

◆ remembering things;

◆ working things out;
◆ learning anything new;
◆ coping with any physical or sensory impairments that develop as a result of normal ageing or the result of illness or accidents;
◆ activities such as finding your way about, driving, and lack of judgement.

These symptoms don't come alone. There will be other issues, depending on what the underlying disease process is, and different symptoms come to the fore at different times. People with dementia often have language problems and their behaviour may change. They might be more irritable than before especially if the environment is noisy or difficult. Families often notice repeated questions, making them seem anxious and finding it difficult to plan. The key problem is a reduction in the person's capacity to do everything. Put together, these symptoms cause phenomenal stress and a crushing fatigue. So it is really important to take the symptoms seriously, even in the very early stages.

I went to the doctor to say I was having problems with calculations, and he laughed and said that I was still better at them than him. I assumed he was just reassuring me with a little pleasantry and that he'd refer me to a specialist but he did nothing. (Retired scientist, 78)

Remembering things
Memory is not the worst for me. I've learned to use a lot of

props – diaries, Post-it notes, electronic things like my ...
What's it called? ... hand phone ... mobile ... What was I
saying? ... [prompted: 'Forgetting?'] Yes ... People think I've
forgotten how to do things ... but it's as if time has gone
funny. I stare at the task for ages and then realise that ten
minutes have passed and I've not done it ... [long pause] ...
I've not forgotten how to do it. I just somehow forget to start
... and then I'm slow. (Early-retired nurse, 57)

There is no doubt that people with dementia have
memory problems. When they lose memories of
past events, it often happens in a characteristic way
where the most recent memories fade fastest. People
may describe a situation in which they can recall the
names of all the players in a sports team from thirty
years ago, but they're not sure if they ate lunch today.
They may remember how to use skills that they learned
in childhood or early adulthood, but more recently
learned things are slipping away from them.

One way this shows up is people going home to the
wrong house – maybe the house they lived in twenty
years ago. They don't 'remember' where they now live.
Another distressing example is failing to recognise close
family members.

Every single time I see my uncle he looks at me as if he is
puzzled and says, 'You've changed. You look different.'
Even if he saw me only the day before ... I've realised now
that his memory of me is fixed about fifteen or twenty
years ago, before my hair and beard started to go grey. He
recognises me, but within twenty-four hours he's forgotten
again that I'm in my fifties and he's still expecting the

thirty-something me when I knock on his door the next morning. (Nephew, 55)

This can be really painful for family members, particularly young ones. As recent additions to the family and the newest additions to the family tree, they are the first to disappear from the story. When you think of the excitement and joy of the birth of a grandchild, and the special relationship with a grandparent, it is almost unbearable that they may one day look at the child or young person and say, 'And who are you, young lady?' You need to think about how you are going to explain this when children ask, 'Does Granny not love me any more? Why doesn't she know me?' There are books which explore these issues sensitively with young people and internationally a number of children's authors set out stories about this in beautifully illustrated and carefully crafted books that you may feel comfortable reading with smaller children (see Helpful organisations and Resources at the end of this book). When the person with dementia makes a mistake like this, they feel embarrassment and shame, or confusion and anger – a whole range of emotions – so think about how to handle conversations in a way that helps to keep things calm. Maintaining a tranquil atmosphere makes a huge difference if you can manage it.

It is even more crushing if your mother or father stops knowing who you are. You arrive at the house and start to bring in the groceries for them and they shout at you and tell you to go away. 'If you don't leave at once I'll get my son to deal with you,' your mother says. 'But I am your son!'

People do really believe that in some sense their mother has died if she does not know them any more and that they are meeting a stranger who inhabits their mother's body. One strategy to try is to ask your mother if she has a daughter or son, and see her face light up as she tells you all about her darling, then remember that, in truth, that's *you*.

There are no rules about how to handle this, except to avoid arguments if possible. A key message is that the person with dementia has worse symptoms if they are facing a lot of challenges. See if you can avoid unnecessary challenges. And there are lots of things that can help with memory difficulties at different stages of the dementia. There is more about this later in the book.

You should see our refrigerator. It is covered with magnets holding notes up for Mom reminding her about stuff. I know that she studies the notes and uses them. I've passed the kitchen door and glanced in to see her with her glasses on the end of her nose, peering at them. (Daughter, 57)

Working things out

Difficulty in working things out is sometimes described as 'loss of executive function'. Not being able to remember things becomes a serious issue if you are unable to undertake this basic function, which normally compensates for memory gaps in most people. Imagine waking up in a hospital bed. It may take a few moments to work out where you are and what to do. There are lots of clues – machines and people in uniforms, and curtains and lockers. You don't remember how you got there, but you've worked out where you are so there are possible explanations. You wonder, 'Did I have an accident?' If the nurse comes and tells you that you were knocked off your bike and hit your head, and that you'll be fine and your son has phoned from work and is on his way to the hospital, then you can relax on your pillows and think, 'Wow! That was a lucky escape.'

Now again imagine waking up not knowing where you are. Nothing round you gives you a clue. There are machines and people in uniforms, and curtains and lockers that remind you of ... what? You can't think. The nurse comes and tells you why you are there, and seconds later you can't remember her or what she said. You decide to get up and explore and you still can't work out where you are. The more you struggle to understand the less sense it makes. You start to wonder if you've been drugged and brought here against your will. Then panic sets in as you realise that your young son must be waiting for you at the school gate. You need to leave. Someone tries to stop you and you fight them and they sedate you.

In both cases there is a memory problem. You can't remember how you got to where you are. In one case you can work it out, and make use of new information presented by the nurse, but in the other you can't, and you dredge up old or even invented bits of information to try to fill the gaps. The first situation becomes more reassuring by the minute, while the second becomes more nightmarish. That second situation is what dementia feels like. It's intensely stressful.

Where am I? Where am I? I am in hell. (Plea from a woman with dementia in an acute hospital, quoted by a hospital visitor)

There are very many activities we do every day on autopilot, but if you break them down they are really complicated executive functions. Just getting out to work, even if you have no family responsibilities, is complex. You need to be organised the night before, and have clean appropriate clothes ready to put on, and in the morning you need to get out of your night-clothes, eat, shower and shave or put on make-up and check your home is secure, before heading off with your travel pass or car keys. If you have lost executive function you may know you have to do these things, but not be able to put it all together. A lady found in the street in her nightclothes has not necessarily 'forgotten' to get dressed. She's just not putting things together as she did every day of her life till now. Because of difficulties in thinking, she is in fact preparing for a day in the past. She's long retired. She has nowhere she needs to go, no matter how overwhelming her sense that she must get up and get on with things. And so she leaves the house before dressing or eating. Insight into how loss of the capacity to work things out and loss of executive function disable people with dementia gives us a clue about how to handle this sort of situation. You can avoid a lot of trouble if you try very hard to get inside the head of the person with dementia. Not trying is the mistake that many professionals make. This lady does not need to be 'put away for her own safety'. She more probably needs some prompting and distracting at the time of day that she is most likely to set off on the wrong track, and that may be not random but the same time every day, making it easier for you to work out how to resolve the problem.

Learning anything new

Being aware of the difficulty with new learning is vital for understanding and managing the problem that people with dementia have of forgetting recent things. When we are children and our brains are developing our parents and teachers rehearse us over and over until knowledge 'sinks in'. Toddlers, who learn when asked, 'What does the dog say?' to reply 'Bow-wow!' know they will be rewarded with laughter and attention. Training humans and animals like pets to respond to a reward is well recognised as a deliberate teaching technique and we use it instinctively with babies. This is a form of operant conditioning, which is a process where behaviour is modified by the consequence of the behaviour. It's an important part of learning. You do something again because of the positive outcome. But what happens if you can't make the connection between what you did and what happens next?

Recently there has been interest in the very small number of children who develop a form of dementia. A good understanding of the limitations of traditional teaching methods is really important for those who are caring for them. Because they are at school, they are in an environment where people are rewarded for new learning, and where teachers go over things again and again until pupils know them. When the child starts to say he does not know what he knew yesterday, he may be suspected of being lazy or wilfully naughty. Parents even get angry and frustrated. The particular children who have the disorders that can be seen as 'dementia' have mostly started life with a learning difficulty in any case, so the disintegration of what they have achieved with so much effort is a double tragedy. Their families have to learn quickly how to cope with this new reality and stop 'rewarding' 'good' behaviour and 'discouraging' the 'wrong' behaviour. What works with other kids is just frustrating and confusing for children with dementia. In caring for adults with dementia we have a great deal to learn from these resourceful families, teachers and paediatricians who are managing a reduction in the capacity to learn in this very small group of children.

Not least, we all need to learn that when we point out that something has not been learned by the person with dementia they will feel shame and anger with themselves. Given that we ought to know that they have problems learning, why would we be so insensitive?

In the hospital, I was talking to the consultant and we were interrupted by the presence of an old man who was clearly busting to ask a question. He was neatly dressed, washed and shaved and very polite. 'Doctor, I'm ready to go now. When am I going home?' The doctor sighed and all but rolled his eyes and said, 'I told you already that will be Friday.' I've never seen such a crestfallen look on anyone's face. The patient wasn't just disappointed, but profoundly embarrassed to discover that he'd already been annoying the

Great Man with his stupid questions. He looked slapped.
Almost immediately he could not remember the exchange
but his sense of discomfort lasted much longer than the
memory of how he'd gone wrong. He retained a profound
reduction in his self-confidence. (Hospital visitor)

Because the person has difficulty with learning new things, it is as if they have forgotten. When the nurse says, 'But I told her where the toilet is and how to use the call button,' she is displaying a lack of understanding. The person with dementia may have forgotten these instructions before the nurse has finished reciting them. They never learned them at the time. We have to ask ourselves why we want this person to learn a new thing, such as how to get the nurse by pressing the button or that they should not press the button every thirty seconds. If reaching a nurse when you need one depends on you learning a new skill under current hospital arrangements, we need to change the hospital arrangements. When up to 50 per cent of hospitalised patients have confusion, why would you equip the staff with a complex, unfamiliar method for their patients to call for help? The person with dementia in these circumstances may find it beyond them to learn to use it properly. It's not impossible to learn new things after diagnosis, but in general this capacity is starting to slip and it will continue to do so over time. It's bizarre that a nurse would describe someone as 'forgetting' something they never learned.

Families can inadvertently reinforce the humiliation of the person with dementia because of their own embarrassment. It can feel as if your relative is 'behaving badly'.

Mother, did you not hear what the doctor said? He is asking you if you have been sleeping well … (Mother ignores both.) Speak up now. Remember what you told me. He won't come and see you again if you don't talk to him … (Mother shouts angrily.) Please don't use that kind of language!! (Son of woman with dementia, during doctor visit)

Coping with physical or sensory impairments

Mother had apparently said to the nurses, 'I can't read.' So when the mobile library went round they just passed her by. Actually she loves to read, and I got her a bright light and some large-print books, and she devoured them. They said to me, 'We actually thought she was not able to read. We did not realise.' They thought it was the dementia. I'm saddened by their ignorance and confusion about dementia because it is her that suffers when THEY get confused. (Daughter of Mary, 85)

It is important to remember that about 5 per cent of people with dementia are of working age. That used to be forgotten. The other 95 per cent are old or very old. All older people will experience the changes of ageing, which usually include physical or sensory impairment. Reading glasses, walking aids and hearing aids are getting less expensive and more sophisticated all the time, so most of us are compensating well. However, if you have a problem with learning new things, you may be unable to use some of the aids that are available. It could be as simple as not remembering to put on your glasses, or failing to eat properly because you have forgotten how to use your dentures.

The loss of confidence that follows as a result of adverse incidents created by these problems can lead to someone not wanting to go out and about any more. The person with dementia has even greater difficulty in adapting to changes in their physical capacity than other older people. For example, if you aren't good at remembering where you are, it is really important for you to be able to see where you are. All older people need more light because of age-related changes in the eye, but if you've got dementia it matters even more. The increased light will help you to see objects you might have forgotten, and gives more information to help you work things out. (See Chapter 9 for ideas on lighting design.) But if you have dementia you may forget to put the light on, or make an unwise decision to economise on power or electricity, not realizing how false that economy would be.

In addition, depending on what the underlying cause of the dementia is, you might have other problems. For example, people with vascular dementia are more likely to have spatial-awareness problems that create a risk that they will fall over. Fear of falling is very debilitating for older people. If they have already fallen and suffered a fracture, the patient with dementia in hospital may not remember that they mustn't try to stand alone while they are undergoing rehabilitation. There is a great temptation under these circumstances to use restraints, like safety straps that tie them to a chair or a bed. But in the end this may cause even more injury as the person tries to escape, having forgotten (or never learned) why they are tied down.

I will never use restraints again, or allow my nurses to use them. I wish I could get them banned altogether. I walked on to the ward one day just as one of the patients had wriggled and wriggled in her seat to try to get out, and she had slipped down and the lap strap was at her throat. Everyone was busy and had not noticed. If I had not walked by at that moment she would have been strangled. (Ward sister)

It is not unusual in some countries to see the use of restraint equipment such as a straightjacket to keep an older person in bed for fear of falling.

In my last trip overseas I was invited by a heroic nurse who had ended the use of restraint for confused elderly people in her own hospital. She wanted me to help raise the issue in other hospitals, to start a change programme. For the first time in my life I saw an agitated old lady tied to the bed. It was a modern, well equipped place, but the cultural norm was to tie people up. Added to that every staff member wore a paper surgical face mask for infection control (a futile policy). It must have been terrifying for the patient. (Experienced dementia nurse)

Finding your way about, driving and lack of judgement

Finding your way about

People with dementia are sometimes described as 'wandering'. Some objections have been raised to using that term because it implies that the person is drifting around for no reason and that they are lost. Curiously, the person is not always lost, but rather looking in a determined and rational way for something which unfortunately is no longer there, or trying to enter a building that no longer belongs to them. They are not lost. It is just that we can't comprehend where they are going, or why.

Our neighbour moved away a short distance, and after, she often came striding along our street staring at each door in turn. We'd go out to meet her, and distract her with conversation and gossip while walking her round the corner to her daughter's house. She kept wandering back to our street, though. (Former neighbour)

It is useful to consider what underlies this problem. Dementia robs people of their most recent memories, so they may forget that they moved to a new house. Or they might be trying to complete something they are thinking of as urgent, long after the need has passed. It is quite common to find old people with dementia looking for and asking for someone, even though they attended that person's funeral years ago. These things happen more often when the person is agitated for another reason, so the advice later in this book about reducing agitation may help with wandering, searching and pacing behaviour.

Driving

Driving is made hazardous for similar reasons. When you learn to drive you pick up some really important skills, such as how to use a roundabout or traffic circle. If you were to travel as the crow flies, you'd never go all the way round to reach your exit. Going the other way, against the traffic, might look quicker and more direct. The person with dementia who decides to take the short route is being perfectly logical, but has forgotten the rules of the road and the danger of ignoring them. Turning right or left into a dual carriageway or divided highway is more complicated than you think. If you've tried to drive in a country where the rules of the road are different from your own, you will know how challenging that is.

Driving requires quick judgement and adherence to regulations, and the person with dementia is slowed in their judgement and has forgotten some of the rules. This is why in many states, regions and countries you are required to tell the vehicle licensing authorities that you have been diagnosed with dementia. You need to check if this is required where you live. Failure to do so might incur penalties and invalidate your insurance, but people are so disabled by losing their car that they are tempted to avoid revealing their news. Doctors who have to be involved in these decisions find it very hard.

In the end we had to take the car away from the house, so even Mom could not use it. While it was there, Dad used to threaten her to get the keys, and drive off. He was so angry. When he first was diagnosed he had a driving test and they let him drive for quite a while after that, but eventually he failed the test. It is really hard, but I'd rather that he was angry with us than that we were explaining to someone why he had run over their child at a crossing point. (Son of Roger, 79)

In some countries such as Australia you can get a provisional permit that allows you to drive in a restricted area, as long as someone is with you in the vehicle. It may be frustrating to go back to being like a learner, but in reality, with dementia, you become more 'inexperienced' as a driver with the passage of time as the recent memories and skills fade. There is no such scheme at present in the United States or Canada, even in remote or rural areas where it works best.

In the United States there are resources that can be accessed to help with this difficult problem through the AARP (www.aarp.org) and the Association for Driver Rehabilitation Specialists (www.aded.net). The National Highway Traffic Safety Administration (www.nhtsa.gov) also has useful advice on what if any requirements each State's Department of Motor Vehicles (DMV) requires in terms of monitoring drivers with dementia. Some DMVs have staff who are trained in recognizing impairments in older adults. The State law may not refer specifically to Alzheimer's disease but may mention cognitive impairment, or mental disease or impairment. Reports to the DMV can be made by a relative or concerned citizen, as well as a medical professional. The variation in driving regulations and tests from State to State has given rise to speculation that drivers might relocate to places with less stringent rules, which would be a particularly dangerous practice. Relocation in itself carries risks for people with cognitive impairment. The

Hartford Financial Services Group, Inc., and the MIT AgeLab have developed a guide to help people with dementia and their families prolong independence while encouraging safe driving. The guide provides suggestions for monitoring, limiting and stopping driving. The information incorporates the experiences of family caregivers and people with dementia, as well as suggestions from experts in medicine, gerontology and transportation. (http://hartfordauto.thehartford.com/UI/Downloads/Crossroads.pdf)

I'll be fine. My daughter worries about me, I know, but I have no idea what I'd do without the car. I don't want to be dependent. (James, 87)

In Canada you can get up-to-date advice from the Alzheimer Society of Canada who provide a Driving and Dementia tip sheet on their website at www.alzheimer.ca.

The advice of Alzheimer's Australia makes it clear that all drivers in Australia are required by law to tell their local licensing authority about dementia – a doctor's assessment follows and then perhaps a formal driving assessment.

If the person with dementia can continue to drive they will be issued a conditional license. Conditional licenses are valid for a maximum of 12 months; after that the driver will be reassessed. Sometimes restrictions are also placed on the license holder. These restrictions might be that the person can only drive close to home, at certain times, or below certain speed limits. (Alzheimer's Australia)

You must check the regulations in your own country, state or region, in case the insurance or licence is invalidated by dementia, but remember that a driving ban is not automatic at the early stages when the person is still quite well.

It was really hard getting dad to give up driving, but we talked about it a lot in advance and looked at alternatives, like getting stuff delivered, and rallying round to keep him on the move. (Daughter)

Lack of judgement

Lack of judgement is a complicated thing to assess. If a person who was always averse to risk starts to do things they'd never have done before, is that them losing their judgement, or are they just starting to 'live a little'? It would be wrong to restrict someone who wants to have an adventure, or be creative, but at times we have a duty of care.

Mom decided that she was going to remove the overhanging branches from a high tree in her garden. I've never seen her up a ladder in her life, but she was dragging it up the path, with an axe in her other hand. I distracted her and hid the ladder and axe where she'll never find them but she's mad at me. She does not remember why ... but she still wants to remove those branches. (Daughter)

The daughter made her judgement and acted. There are no rules for this sort of thing, which is what makes dementia such a complicated and difficult issue.

Not least, the person with dementia is a prime target

for financial fraud. The AARP Fraud Watch Network in the USA gives access to information about how to stay up on the con artists' latest tricks and what to do. You don't have to be an AARP member to access it. At the end of 2015 they launched an education programme to help people avoid identity theft. Simple things can make a difference, such as locking your mailbox, carefully destroying obsolete personal documents and never giving out personal information unless you know who is asking for it and why they need it. People with dementia might not exercise the judgement needed to do all of this.

Stress

All of the symptoms outlined here (difficulties with remembering, working things out, learning, coping, poor judgement and problems finding your way) give rise to dreadful stress. It is stress that explains some of the dementia-related disturbing behaviour that families and professionals find hard to understand.

I got into trouble from the nurse for calling what Ethel was doing 'disturbing'. Well, I don't know what the right language is but she certainly disturbed me. The nurse says that all Ethel is doing is expressing distress because of all the stress she is experiencing. She says calling it 'disturbed' behaviour is wrong. (I'll call it what I like when the nurse is gone ... I'm a bit stressed myself.) (Home care worker for Ethel, 92)

The more challenging the environment is for people with dementia, the more stress they and those around them will suffer. The main challenges have been identified by research. They include the behaviour of other people, the hazards in the physical environment in terms of noise and light, and the design of spaces. Another challenge is presented when the person is required to go through rapid change and faces too many people and new systems and processes. The person may already be undermined physically by poor diet, lack of exercise and even dehydration, on top of whatever cocktail of medicines they have to take for their other ailments. Any intervention that can be made to reduce stress will certainly make life easier, both for the person with dementia and for the family caregiver.

What are the different diseases that can cause these symptoms?

Alzheimer's disease

Alzheimer's disease is the most common cause of dementia and probably over 47.5 million people worldwide are affected by this. Seen through a microscope, abnormal clumps appear in the brain tissue, along with tangled fibres that should not be there. There is a loss of connection between brain cells, which eventually die. It is clear that the brain damage starts long before there are any behavioural symptoms. A person might not ever have had dementia symptoms in their lifetime, but might be found to have changes in their brain tissue caused by Alzheimer's disease at a post-mortem examination. As an affected person gets older, more brain cells die and whole regions of the brain start to shrink so unmistakably that you can see it on simple brain scans. The cause of the disease is not fully understood and that hampers ongoing efforts to find a possible cure. It mainly affects old or very old people, and the older you are the more likely you are to be affected.

Of course, families wonder if it is inherited. The position is complicated. Families who have a record of living to a great age include lots of relatives who lived long enough to get dementia.

Well, the doctor says I'm getting the dementia now and I am celebrating. I'm ninety-six, you know, and I did not die in an accident or from cancer or in the war, and I've still most of my teeth (enough anyway) and something has to get you in the end. It's OK. All my brothers and sisters lived to be over ninety and I was the youngest. It's just my time. Two of them had it, but not bad. (Retired schoolteacher)

Recent studies have started looking at what we now call the 'Fourth Age'. This term is used to classify people over eighty-five. They are extreme survivors. It is as if those of us under that age are still being 'weeded out', but if you make it to eighty-five you may be around for much longer and are probably really tough in a way that is worth studying.

If you are unfortunate enough to be in a family where anyone got Alzheimer's disease before they were sixty years old, then your family is possibly affected by a dementia that has more genetic factors than the others. One contribution to the lack of knowledge about family connections in the past was the stigma that used to surround any mental health problem. Someone with 'early-onset' 'young onset' or 'working-age' dementia these days will sometimes reveal that one of their parents did die young, but no one ever talked to them about the cause of death, and it was swept under the carpet so they didn't know much about it as children, and now no one is alive who knew. Many people in these families will never inherit the dementia, though, and it is important to ask your doctor for genetic counselling if worry about this is affecting your life.

In Alzheimer's disease the causes of the plaques and tangles are still to be worked out. The amount of time and money spent on Alzheimer's disease research has increased in recent years. President Obama in the United States supported a 'We Can't Wait' initiative planning huge increases in research investment. Dementia is so expensive to society and so feared that there will be great prizes and financial rewards for anyone who can find a cure. Cruelly, there are press stories nearly every week about the latest breakthrough, but on closer reading they are usually unconvincing. The increases in research money announced in the UK are from a very low level – only a fraction of what is spent on cancer research. This is ironic when you realise that in that country dementia costs more than cancer, heart disease and stroke put together: around £23 billion (US$35 billion) was spent on dementia in 2012. How much is spent in other countries may be harder to determine, without really knowing how many people have been diagnosed. The United States around the same time was presumed to be spending over $200 billion, not including the cost to families and family caregivers. There is probably a huge amount of additional hidden expense as people with dementia who have not been diagnosed get caught up in health and social care systems.

A number of years ago when it was reported in the newspapers that there were high levels of aluminium in abnormal Alzheimer's disease brain tissue, people threw out all their metal pots and pans and bought glass ones. That was pointless, because we get aluminium in our diet anyway from a range of other sources, including indigestion remedies, but it illustrates how people react to single 'research discovery' stories in the news. It is ironic that the evidence that exercise makes a difference has been building up all the time, but you don't always see that coming through on health education messages. We don't see people throwing away their sofa to avoid memory loss ... but all of us ought to be sitting down less.

The important thing to remember about Alzheimer's disease is that it's a gradual process that starts years before any symptoms set in. So if you know someone has Alzheimer's disease and their dementia symptoms suddenly become very much worse, it is unlikely that the Alzheimer's disease process is causing this sudden deterioration. It's more likely that they've got some other illness brewing, like an infection or a delirium. If they are treated, the person can go back towards their previous level of functioning.

This retired teacher with Alzheimer's disease was living well at home in the house she had occupied for fifty years, just having daily visits from the daughter. She was discovered fallen one day and taken to hospital, where she was diagnosed with a urinary tract infection and started on antibiotics, but unfortunately she had a fall while in hospital when she confused the location of the toilet and fractured her hip. Rehabilitation was slow and she became disturbed and was judged unfit to return home, having failed a kitchen assessment with the OT (occupational therapy) staff. Care home destination was recommended. In the care home she was agitated and aggressive and antipsychotic medication was prescribed, and shortly after this she had a stroke and died. It is my view that if the urinary tract infection had been treated at home this lady would be alive today. We could have tried harder. (Specialist dementia nurse)

In Alzheimer's disease it is particularly valuable to have an early diagnosis because there is some Alzheimer's-specific medication that can help, and you can't access that till you've been diagnosed. Also, it works best in the early stages, so you don't want to miss that window of opportunity. There are lifestyle changes that you can make to significantly reduce the symptoms, even though they don't alter the disease process a lot. They are worthwhile because they make the journey easier, and some of them are enjoyable in their own right. But the medication is time-sensitive, so you want to access it at the right time.

The organisations in each country of the world which support people with dementia and their caregivers are almost universally known as 'Alzheimer's' organisations, a convention that has sprung up because in many languages the word 'dementia' has offensive connotations. Although called 'Alzheimer's', they take an interest in other non-Alzheimer's types of dementia, and want to influence policies that will affect all causes of dementia. Those organisations, supported by over-arching organisations like Alzheimer's Disease International (ADI) and Alzheimer Europe, have played an important part in raising political awareness of dementia. One of the most helpful tools in their work is the increasing amount of evidence about the financial cost of dementia to society, and their prediction that numbers affected are going to double in the next twenty years. In any country it may be that the finance minister has as much interest in this as the health minister. This is why former UK Prime Minister David Cameron chose dementia as the theme for a G8 summit in 2013. It's a huge issue.

There are a couple of good reasons for emphasizing the linguistic point. When the media gets excited about 'developments in treatment' or 'cures' for 'Alzheimer's disease' (or 'AD') it is important to question whether they really mean Alzheimer's, or if they are referring to all forms of dementia. The truth is that even if we did have a way of preventing Alzheimer's disease today a lot of other people would still develop dementia symptoms, because they had been harbouring the disease for decades or because their particular dementia was not caused by Alzheimer's. And the search for the cure for other causes of dementia would still need to go on.

Vascular disease

This is the second most common cause of dementia. The problem here is the blood supply to the brain. The symptoms generally come on more suddenly than in Alzheimer's disease. It may happen after a stroke or a series of strokes. What makes vascular dementia like a stroke is that both are caused by problems with the blood supply, as a result of which a bit of brain tissue dies. The Australian dementia organisations coined a great phrase: 'What's good for your heart is good for your head.' Any health problems that are likely to cause difficulties with circulation and increase the risk of heart attack will increase the risk of vascular dementia. This would include high blood pressure, diabetes, high cholesterol and any heart-related problems – and in addition all the lifestyle issues that make those conditions worse: like lack of exercise, smoking and eating too much of the wrong sort of food.

One of the biggest differences between vascular dementia and Alzheimer's dementia lies in the underlying disease process. In Alzheimer's the brain shrinks relatively slowly as individual brain cells die back and so the symptoms creep up over time. In vascular dementia, although this pattern can sometimes be seen, there is often a distinct moment when the blood vessel gets blocked. The person can be stable for a long period and then deteriorate suddenly to a lower level of functioning as another bunch of blood vessels gets blocked by a clot. That's more likely when there is narrowing of the blood vessel caused by thickening of the wall where fat deposits have gathered. The symptoms of vascular dementia depend on which part of the brain has been damaged. The commonest form is called 'multi-infarct' dementia. This is where there are lots of tiny strokes taking out lots of different areas. Each lobe of the brain does a different job and doctors can tell where the damage was from scans. That knowledge can give some insight into what problems you might expect. Deep inside the brain, at what is called the 'subcortical' level, there are tiny blood vessels which can be damaged when the person has a stroke. This is called subcortical vascular dementia (it used to be called Binswanger's disease). The symptoms of that dementia include difficulties in walking, clumsiness, lack of facial expression and speech difficulties. The older someone is, the more likely they are to have a mixture of vascular disease and Alzheimer's. In fact, the older someone is, the more likely that, at autopsy, their brain will show evidence of a large number of the changes that are associated with dementia, even if they didn't seem to have dementia symptoms.

My dad had a small stroke and then declined rapidly over twelve months, and he's in a care home now after his second stroke, but I met a man who told me he has vascular dementia as well and he's living at home. His experience was that he got very bad over a few months and since then he's been stable for three years. It seems that everyone is different. (Son of man with multi-infarct dementia, 72)

Vascular dementia can run in a family if the family has a history of stroke or cardiovascular disease. Indian,

Pakistani, African-American, Afro-Caribbean and Sri Lankan communities have a high prevalence of vascular risk factors and more research needs to be done to see how their risk can be reduced. Vascular dementia is progressive, but treating the underlying medical conditions can help to slow the rate of decline. This includes managing high blood pressure, cholesterol, diabetes or heart problems. There is no recommended drug for vascular dementia itself, unlike Alzheimer's disease, but if the patient has a mixed dementia the Alzheimer's medication may be recommended. However, given the recent emphasis on public health measures like smoking cessation and education about keeping fit, it is interesting that this coincides with a recently detected possible slowing of the numbers being identified with dementia. It is too soon to say that this means we're preventing it, but that would be the logical conclusion. And wonderful, if true.

Dementia with Lewy bodies (Lewy body dementia)

Lewy bodies are tiny lumps of protein in the brain which disrupt normal functioning. No one really knows where they come from or how they do this. Similar abnormal proteins are found also in the brains of people with Parkinson's disease. Unfortunately many people with Parkinson's do go on to develop dementia that resembles the Lewy body type of dementia.

About one in ten people with dementia have this type. It is rare below sixty-five years of age, but not unknown. Because it is rare it is not always spotted and gets mistaken for Alzheimer's disease. The person may get some symptoms of Parkinson's disease, which include loss of facial expression, an inclination to shuffle and limb stiffness. People describe vivid hallucinations.

Dad was kind of rooted in his chair and I was trying to get him to mobilise a bit. I thought the problem was the muscle stiffness, but he said that he was afraid if he stood up he might hurt the little animals that were sitting on the carpet round his chair. (Daughter of Mr B., 67)

In Chapter 7 there is more discussion about what you can do when someone is hallucinating. These symptoms ebb and flow on a daily or hourly basis. It is not unusual for the person to doze a lot during the day and then have agitated nights troubled by hallucinations and nightmares. They will have falls and fainting attacks. That combination of fluctuation and hallucinations is what will lead the doctor to think that it is the Lewy body type of dementia.

Lewy body disease is the prime example of why it is useful to know what the underlying cause of the dementia is. It is not unusual for a person with dementia to exhibit disturbing behaviour. It is regrettably not unusual for them to be prescribed antipsychotic medication in a rather slapdash approach as an attempt to tranquillize them. These are also known as 'neuroleptics', or 'major tranquilizers'.

The message here is that antipsychotics should only be used in very specific circumstances in order to treat psychotic symptoms and never used just for the sedative effect (which is often called a 'chemical restraint'). By 'psychotic'

symptoms I mean delusions and hallucinations which
are so disturbing for the patient that you really need to
do something to help them. If you prescribe them at all
it should be done with extreme caution in dementia with
Lewy bodies and Parkinson's disease. I'm tempted almost
to say 'never' in Lewy body disease. (Dr Cesar Rodriguez,
Consultant Old Age Psychiatrist)

Even where there are no serious side effects, this medication often does not work and yet it continues to be administered despite the fact that it is extremely dangerous and can cause strokes or other fatal complications. But in Lewy body dementia specifically there is a particular risk from antipsychotics that will reduce life expectancy and cause very disturbing side effects that are irreversible if you don't catch them early.

Our aunt was admitted to a care home where they told me
she was 'resistive to care', whatever that means, and they
put her on some medication and she just stopped. I mean
she stopped walking, and eating. She lay on her bed and
was as stiff as a board. It was like she was dying. [A friend]
... recommended that I ask them for a list of her medication
and they refused that day, but the next day they gave me
one. I did not understand but it was very short. They said
they'd had the doctor in and he had reduced some stuff.
She started to get better almost at once. She is her old self.
(Nephew of retired schoolteacher, 80)

It appears that by asking the question about medication this family had alerted the staff and prompted them to get it checked, even though the family didn't understand the list when it came. Perhaps the doctor stopped the antipsychotic medicine when it was drawn to his attention that someone was checking. You can always check out a list of medications with a pharmacist – for example the community pharmacist at your local drug store or pharmacy. They are astonishingly smart and they love to look for medicines that you shouldn't take because of something else you have wrong with you and medicines that don't mix well. Your pharmacist is your friend. A list of the names of some of those dangerous medicines might help, but names change and the same medicine can have more than one name even in one country. This is because each company that produces it can give its own product a name in addition to the generic name, which is called the 'proprietary' name.

Isolated dementia with Lewy bodies (DLB) is relatively uncommon. It is much more usual to find a mixture of DLB and Alzheimer's disease, especially in patients who are over 70 years of age. The patients with the best response to the medication we call cholinesterase inhibitors usually have that mixture of both DLB and Alzheimer's disease. (Professor Kenneth Rockwood, Kathryn Allen Weldon Professor of Alzheimer's Research, Dalhousie University, Halifax, Nova Scotia)

In the UK the drugs for Alzheimer's are not 'licensed' for use in patients with Lewy body dementia, but they are sometimes used with good effect. Licensing a drug means approving it formally for a particular type of patient. In using them outside of the licence, the doctor is taking a calculated risk in the belief that it will benefit the patient.

Frontotemporal dementia

This is the name given to a range of conditions including Pick's disease and the dementia that can come with motor neuron disease. These conditions are grouped together because the part of the brain affected in each case is the area responsible for behaviour, emotions and language, and so the problems that the person has may be similar in each case. The brain gets a build-up of abnormal proteins, as seen in Alzheimer's disease, so that brain cells are progressively lost and the affected area of the brain shrinks. It is unusual for someone to develop this when they are over the age of 80.

In the days when we had double rooms there was a family that asked for their grandmother to be moved out because she had started to use some really quite choice foul language. They thought she was picking it up from the other lady. It was quite a delicate job explaining that it was the dementia. As the front lobe of her brain was damaged all the proper manners and inhibitions that she had as a proper lady were breaking down, and it wasn't anyone's fault, but the disease. (Care home manager)

Although this is the tale of an older person, frontotemporal dementia is a greater cause of dementia in those under the age of sixty-five, where it is the second most common cause after early-onset Alzheimer's disease. Almost half of cases have a family history of the disease, so there has been some progress in identifying the relevant genes that are causing the problems. Genes act as chemical instructions inside cells, which allow the body to make things, and if they go wrong that gives rise to problems. Some of those problems can be passed down in families because you inherit your genes from your parents, but in the other cases it is not known what causes this frontotemporal dementia. The person's behaviour and their personality alter for the worse, which is very distressing for families as the person lacks insight and loses the capacity to identify with others. They appear to become self-centred and insensitive and they may even fall foul of the law. Because the patients are younger, facilities and services are less likely to be geared up for their needs and so having a proper diagnosis goes some way towards giving a family a strategy for living with this problem.

People think of my husband as being a rather difficult, nasty, rude person, which he never ever was before. He loses his temper and annoys other people. Our children can't bring their friends to the house because he says inappropriate things. (Wife of man with frontotemporal dementia)

The top tips about dementia knowledge and awareness

◆ Be aware that a lot of the people you meet in professional jobs may not always have an in-depth understanding of dementia.

◆ With Alzheimer's dementia there is some medication available to temporarily delay the disease processes, but otherwise treatment is all about symptom control and keeping well.

◆ You can find out a great deal about the sort of dementia that is affecting you or your family, but first you need a diagnosis.

chapter 2

Getting a diagnosis

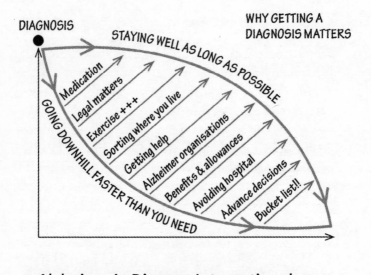

DIAGNOSIS

WHY GETTING A
DIAGNOSIS MATTERS

STAYING WELL AS LONG AS POSSIBLE

Medication

Legal matters

Exercise +++

Sorting where you live

Getting help

Alzheimer organisations

Benefits & allowances

Avoiding hospital

Advance decisions

Bucket list!!

GOING DOWNHILL FASTER THAN YOU NEED

Alzheimer's Disease International

This world-wide federation of Alzheimer associations works tirelessly to support people with dementia across the world and their recommendations are quite clear, including the following:

◆ Every country should have a national dementia strategy promoting early diagnosis.

◆ All primary care services should have basic skills in diagnosis and initial management.

◆ Professionals need to know what drug and non-drug interventions work.

The fact that they had to say this in 2011 illustrated that it was not already happening, but it is getting better all the time.

Are you worried about your memory?

People worry about whether or not they have dementia yet avoid trying to find out. It is vital to get a diagnosis – and not only because there are some conditions that look like dementia which respond really well to treatment. Facing the problem is the first step towards getting help. This chapter looks at how hard it can be to get a diagnosis and how to help someone (or yourself) through that process. The most important message to give people is that it is never too soon to see your doctor if you are worried that you might have dementia and equally it is never too late. So when should you worry?

I wish there was some advice on how to raise the issue with someone? And how to support them through the trauma of a memory test? We never asked my mother, which means that seven years on, the one person who has had no input into decisions about her care … is Mom. And I really don't think we are unusual. (Ruth, whose mother was affected by dementia)

Ordinary forgetting

All of us forget stuff from time to time. Some people habitually forget names or are always losing bits of paper or keys. The important words here are 'habitually' and 'always'. Even though you have always been scatterbrained, you may become self-conscious about it only when you are older. You might worry that others will comment on it. How you do at maths, or map-reading, may get worse as you get older. The time to worry about dementia is when you start to get very much worse. What your family and friends notice is important, so ask them. Did I used to get mixed up like this? With luck, they'll laugh and give you even worse examples from your own past. You are not getting worse. That is just ordinary forgetting. There is also an element of slowing down. The older you get the more answers you will know in the pub quiz, but the younger ones will get their answers out faster than you. That's annoying and so a good reason for having a mix of ages in the team.

Dementia is not ordinary forgetting. It is ordinary to forget phone numbers. It is more worrying if you start to forget how to use a phone or what it is for. Dementia is when you have a marked reduction in your capacity to both remember and do things. If you were great at maths or map-reading you may slow down, but you should still be able to do it. If maths just doesn't make sense any more and you are holding the map upside-down or getting cross and throwing it away, it is worth thinking about seeing someone.

There is no such thing as 'normal' memory. Everyone is different. The most important concern is if you've had a progressive downhill change from what is 'normal' for you. Some people advise that you should have reached the stage where it is causing real problems in your life before thinking it might be dementia. The difficulty with this is that what causes a problem for you actually depends more on your resources than the severity of the symptoms.

Dad was reluctant to drive after he got lost a couple of times and had some scrapes trying to park and so we got him an account with a local taxi firm and he is fine now. (Daughter of 75-year-old man)

Getting your dad a chauffeur service stops the driving problem, but in case the driving problem was a sign that something major was going wrong it is worth getting him to check it out. The doctor would want to know if he's having other problems, like difficulty in following conversations, or trouble performing other familiar tasks, like changing the discs in his DVD player that he learned to use perfectly in the last few years, or managing the ATM cash point machine or using the TV remote control.

Eleanor rammed her bus pass into the ATM to try to get cash out. When I went to speak to the bank counter staff they pointed out icily that this was the fourth or fifth time it had happened over the last two months. (Sister of retired shop worker)

If you are a member of the family and you are asked

by someone if you think they're affected, don't make light of it if you yourself have concerns. Be practical and down to earth.

My brother said that he worried about his memory, so we went for a walk and talked about it together. I asked him what was happening. He described how he'd been driving home recently and found himself parking outside the old house where we used to live. He was always going upstairs to get something and by the time he got there he couldn't remember what he was going for. I pointed out to him that he'd asked me a couple of times recently for money he thought I was due to give him which I thought I'd already given. He was mortified and so was I. I had been too embarrassed to say something at the time. I tried to make him laugh by pretending to complain how he never forgets giving me money but only forgets when I've given it back. Then seriously I suggested that we go and talk to his doctor about it. I went with him. (N., 68)

If you are worried it is a good idea to talk to someone who knows you well to see if they have noticed a change. They might be too embarrassed to say, so even if they give you reassurance it is sensible to mention the problem to the doctor anyway. Write down the concerns you have. A diary is useful to help give a clear picture. It also helps you get a picture for yourself about what is happening.

Is it really dementia?

Some people don't want to raise dementia with their

doctor because they are afraid. They think that there is nothing to be done. They think that if it is bad news they just don't want to know. To be honest, it is always better if you go for the check-up. Some of the symptoms that look like dementia are reversible. It could be that you are coming down with something else, like depression or an infection. Because these are easily treated, it would be a mistake not to see about them and get back to normal as soon as possible. Don't just think it's your age.

He's a work colleague and we are together a lot and I've known him for years. The other day when I was telling someone about him I could not remember his name. I'd been saying how good he was and recommending him and I'm sure the other person thought I was talking rubbish. How could you recommend someone if you don't even know them well enough to remember their name? How true were the stories about our successful joint projects in the light of that? I used to be great at this. Now I find myself going round in circles. It's been for the last six months. (Professor, 58)

There is a long list of things that can affect your memory that are NOT dementia:

◆ loss, such as the death of someone, a divorce or job loss;

◆ nervous tension or worry;

◆ noise or other distractions;

◆ general medicines, particularly if you are taking more than four;

◆ overuse of alcohol;

◆ poor health;

◆ sadness and depression;

◆ side effects of sleeping pills or other sedatives;

◆ sleep deprivation;

◆ some infections, particularly in older people (chest infections and urine infections are notorious);

◆ the menopause;

◆ thyroid disorders;

◆ too many things on your mind;

◆ vitamin B12 deficiency.

Ordinary forgetting can arise for any of these reasons. Are you stressed and tired? Could you be depressed? Some women find that the hormone changes of menopause cause psychological difficulties as well as physiological ones. Have you just got too many things to worry about?

However, if it really is dementia then catching it at the earliest stage is a huge advantage. There is medication that can help in some cases, and you can start to put strategies in place that will let you live a happy life at home for as long as possible.

What should you do?

You should start with your doctor, but don't assume you'll be heard at first. Even though the UK health departments have been saying for years that early diagnosis is really important, in some parts of the UK you've got only a 20 per cent chance of being diagnosed. There is huge variation. In some places it is over 70 per cent. If you don't get a diagnosis, you don't have an explanation for the difficulties you are experiencing. It also excludes you from being offered medication, or accessing any of the support that is outlined in this book. Research shows that many doctors dismiss anxieties until it is too late to undertake some of the really helpful interventions. Of course dementia is very complicated and a family doctor may only see one or two cases a year, so it is not easy. However, more disturbingly, it appears that some doctors are so certain that there is nothing that can be done about dementia, that they think you should not be given a diagnosis because it is of no use to you. This idea can be seen in many other parts of the world. What should you say to get his or her attention? What should you do if he or she seems not to be listening?

I took this daughter to see the doctor who had not tried to diagnose the dementia in her mother for two years, even though everyone in the family and the old lady were quite sure that something was up. I showed him all the local services that were in place that would have helped and the calculation of how many benefits this family had missed out on as a result of her not getting a diagnosis earlier. Over the two years they were nearly £16,000 worse off. He was shocked and pointed out he did not have access to this sort of information, and I told him he only needed to remember one thing: the phone number of the local advocacy organisations, where people were waiting to help families with these sorts of problems. No one was trying to attack him and we've still got a good professional relationship. He tells his colleagues. But I don't have time to visit every doctor in the land. (Age UK manager)

From Argentina, Armenia and Aruba to Venezuela and Zimbabwe, there are Alzheimer organisations throughout the world. These are non-profit associations that support people with dementia and their caregivers, and they are listed on the website of ADI (Alzheimer's Disease International) (www.alz.co.uk) which truly is international even though the HQ is in Europe, in London.

ADI is a good source of advice about what to do initially. They advise that if you're unsure whether you or a loved one may be experiencing the signs or symptoms of Alzheimer's disease, they have a 'Patient/Caregiver Questionnaire' which may help to inform your decision about when it's time to make an appointment with a doctor. Communicating with your doctor is not always easy and they recommend using a journal to track daily behaviour, indications of memory loss, medication use and other important information to help prepare and effectively communicate with your doctor. Recording information on daily routines and bringing it to the next doctor's visit allows the doctor to assess behavioural patterns and identify potential symptoms, which can be difficult to describe during the visit. Alzheimer's Australia has a checklist which can indicate if it is time to visit a doctor.

Many doctors will be interested and motivated to discuss this issue with you. Ask them for a longer appointment because you'll be doing a lot of talking and listening. People worried about dementia in themselves or someone they know should be able to discuss their concerns and the option of seeking a diagnosis with someone who has knowledge and expertise. In your local health system there may be a specialist nurse or psychologist who does this. That is always a good option in my experience. They are specialists themselves and might have even more time for you, but this option is more common in European countries. You need to take time and get information so that you can make an informed decision about what you are going to do next. In some health systems diagnosis is done by a neurologist. The extent to which a neurologist can give advice on activities of daily living varies widely. You can also get advice from dementia expert nurses who practice independently in the United States.

In this area we've got a clinic run by a specialist nurse called Eddie. The doctors can ask patients to make an appointment with him and he'll see them either at the surgery or in their own homes. Eddie says it is actually better in the house. (Alzheimer's Society adviser, UK)

Increasingly health authorities around the world are creating local dementia guidelines and they should know how to put you in touch with someone knowledgeable with whom you can have this sort of discussion. It might be that before going to the doctor you already had a chat with someone else, like a voluntary group or the manager of another service, like a care home, where the person who might have dementia is living.

The Alzheimer Society can help you by providing informa-tion, resources, education, support and counselling.

Also check out our Stories of hope to read about inspirational people who are making a difference in the search for a cure for Alzheimer's disease and other dementias.

Check out your local Alzheimer Society to find out about local programmes and services. (Alzheimer Society of Canada web information)

But it is the doctor (or that specialist nurse) who is the gatekeeper for further diagnostic services in most cases.

People from minority ethnic groups in any country sometimes have difficulty in getting access to good health care. This problem sometimes seems to be even worse if dementia care is needed. If you come from a culture that has a different view of dementia from the mainstream health and social services, it will be hard to get the help you need. This is an issue that needs to be addressed. In the United States, Alzheimer's disease is more prevalent among African-Americans than among whites – with estimates ranging from 14 per cent to almost 100 per cent higher. There is a greater familial risk of Alzheimer's in African-Americans, and because genetic and environmental factors may work differently to cause Alzheimer's disease in African-Americans there have been calls for specific research in this area. A Kaiser Permanente study in the US showed that incidence of dementia was much higher in Native Americans and African-Americans with diabetes than Asian-Americans with diabetes. So there is a complex range of issues involved. And more research is needed.

In late 2015, the Banner Alzheimer's Institute in Arizona hosted the inaugural national conference on this subject in Native American Communities. They said:

The incidence of Alzheimer's disease and related dementias (ADRD) among Native Americans is largely unknown and many tribes lack vocabulary to describe dementia. For more than a decade, the BAI Native American Program has been working with urban and tribal health and social service professionals, family caregivers and communities to increase awareness and care of elders affected by Alzheimer's disease and dementia. (Banner Alzheimer's Institute)

Caregivers in different communities have different views about whether services should be culturally specific or mixed. There are some very successful groups for specific national communities or communities brought together by language or religious faith. In general mainstream services in parts of Europe, for example, people from black and minority ethnic backgrounds are so few that they are clearly not accessing the services. From the statistics we know they exist, but they are missing out on help. In a system where users have to 'fit in' they have a double jeopardy. It's hard to fit in with the mainstream system that may not be culturally sensitive to you and, in any case, people with dementia find it hard to fit in at the best of times.

What happens at the doctor's?

Doctors often do a short mental test in their consulting room. They are sometimes so focused on getting the outcome they don't realise that it can be humiliating to 'fail' the test.

Mum refused to answer. It was as if the test had been designed for her to fail and she would not put herself in that position. (Daughter of 86-year-old woman)

In addition to doing a basic dementia test by asking some questions, the doctor will focus on your general health. Because there are so many reversible physical conditions that might be causing your problem, the doctor will probably recommend blood tests to check:

◆ vitamin B12 and folates;

◆ thyroid function;

◆ minerals, like potassium and calcium;

◆ glucose;

◆ liver and kidney functions;

◆ other routine elements, like counting the blood cells, checking for inflammation.

You might be asked for a urine specimen to see if you've got an infection in your bladder. Older people are different from younger people when they have a urine infection. Younger people complain about itching and burning and needing to run to the bathroom. Older people sometimes just start to seem confused. (The hazard is if health workers assume that all old people are expected to be confused and don't test for and tackle the underlying infection that's causing it.) You might be sent for a chest X-ray if it looks like you've got a chest infection, or for a heart trace (ECG) to see if there is a problem there.

The doctor, if he or she thinks it could be dementia, may send you to a memory assessment service or memory clinic, which can be provided by specialists at the hospital or from a community mental health team.

The US Preventive Services Task Force, a non-governmental panel of health experts, believes that testing in clinically symptomatic older individuals is important. They advise that people with a family member who needs more help with tasks that they have always been able to do should consider scheduling a visit to discuss this with the person's doctor. Under the Affordable Care Act, Medicare in the USA now reimburses people for Annual Wellness Visits that can include an assessment of cognitive function. At the time of writing more than half the people with dementia in the USA don't have a diagnosis.

In some countries when the doctor sends you for further tests you will be attending 'psychiatric' clinics. Part of the problem of asking for help for many people is the stigma about psychiatry and suspicion of those who provide psychiatric services. Don't be put off if you are sent to see someone with 'psychiatry' in their job title. You need to bite the bullet. Memory assessment services come under a variety of names but they specialise in the diagnosis and initial management of dementia and are intended to be the single point of referral for people with a possible diagnosis of dementia. It could be that you see a neurologist.

Your own family doctor or GP ought to know and understand the process of making referrals. They might decide that you've not got a problem that needs to be taken to the specialist clinic right now but that it would make sense to see you again in a while to assess how you are getting on and if things are becoming worse. If you think your concerns are being dismissed, you can ask for a second opinion.

What should happen at the memory assessment service or memory clinic?

Then Mum went to the memory clinic. The day was very long and boring for her, and she did not like it much. But my friend has told me it depends what doctor you get. She and her mum saw a really nice one. And for them a lot of the tests were actually done at home. (Daughter of 86-year-old woman)

Basically you will be asked (or should be) if you want to know the diagnosis once they have made it and who you want to share it with. Usually the assessment will include:

◆ taking a history – that is, asking you all about what has made you go to your doctor with your current problems;

◆ cognitive and mental state examination – that is, a test to see how well your brain is working;

◆ physical examination (that's what doctors do!);

◆ review of medication – that is, seeing if it is your pills that are causing the problem.

It's recommended that if you might have dementia but it is mild and they are not quite sure, they do further 'formal neuropsychological testing'. This means more sets of tests that are used to diagnose brain deficits and usually this will involve a one-to-one conversation in an office. There is a wide range of tests that can be used, but they focus on the areas of memory, orientation, language and problem solving.

... the consultant's conversation with Mum (who is American-born and still has her accent):
Consultant: Well I detect that you might have a bit of an American accent. Can you tell me who is the president of the United States?
Mum: (looking blank) No, I don't think I can remember that.
Consultant: (in a desperate attempt to tap into Mum's longer-term memory) Can you remember which president was assassinated?
Mum: No, I don't.
Consultant: (by now desperately trying to give clues) He had Irish connections.
Mum: (face lighting up with sudden enlightenment) Oh, you mean O'BAMA!
(www.alzheimers.org.uk online forum, 24 March 2013)

At the same time, they'll also want to check if you have any other medical or psychiatric problems that are making your dementia worse. It's not unusual for people diagnosed with dementia to be depressed and everyone needs to keep an eye out for that, because it can be treated. Some people claim that antidepressant medication does not work with people with dementia any more than giving them a bit of support and being sensitive to their feelings. And the last risk you need is any unnecessary pills.

As highlighted in Chapter 1, where different sorts of dementia were described, it is very important to know what 'subtype' of dementia you have: that is, which disease is causing your symptoms.

The doctor says mom has dementia, but she does not have Alzheimer's disease. I don't know what the difference is …
(daughter of Anya, 79)

If the daughter knows what is going on, she'll be more able to understand what might happen next, and not be taken by surprise. This differentiation is best done by specialist staff using evidence-based criteria. It is relatively unusual for them to ask for examination of your spinal fluid, which they do through a lumbar puncture, or spinal tap, but it may happen if you volunteer to take part in research. Sometimes if it is suspected that you have a rapidly progressing form of dementia such as CJD (Creutzfeldt-Jakob disease) or that you might have another disease that can be treated, they will be able to tell that from spinal fluid drained off with a lumbar puncture. In general, EEGs (electroencephalographs or brain traces) are not used for diagnosis but might be considered when there have been epileptic fits, which sometimes come with certain sorts of dementia. They also might recommend a brain trace if there is suspected delirium, frontotemporal dementia or CJD.

MRI (magnetic resonance imaging) and CT (computerised tomography) brain scans are used to help early diagnosis and to detect subcortical changes in blood vessels, where blood vessels deep in the brain have been affected. These scans give good views of the underlying structure and anatomy of the brain. If the person had a previous learning disability the interpretation of these scans is difficult, but earlier diagnosis is getting better all the time.

In the US, amyloid PET scanning may be used for screening. It is expensive, though, and not yet proven as a screening method. In Canada that technology is used only as an investigative tool.

My dad got almost perfect scores on the tests – even though he clearly had a serious problem. The doctor says that because his cognitive starting point was really high – he was a maths professor at an Ivy League University – that meant his scores were really high. The crucial thing was seeing how they had dropped. (Daughter of Prof. A, 86)

Sometimes the family are concerned because the person who seems to have dementia will not be persuaded to see a doctor. If you can find others who have gone through the same situation in your own area it may help. In Australia you can call the National Dementia Helpline on 1800 100 500. In New Zealand there is a Needs Assessment and Service Coordination service (NASC) but in any country the national Alzheimer's organisation may be able to give you the advice that you need, if the doctor does not.

What if it is dementia?

At the clinic someone should take time to discuss the diagnosis with the patient and their family (if the patient agrees). It's recommended that written information is provided on the following:

◆ signs and symptoms;
◆ the course of the disease and what to expect in the future;
◆ treatments that are available if any;
◆ local care and support services;
◆ support groups;
◆ how to stay well;
◆ sources of financial advice;
◆ legal advice and advocacy;
◆ medico-legal issues, such as driving;
◆ local information resources.

Staff want to see if there are any interventions they can use that will help the cognitive symptoms (remembering, working things out ... all the mental functions) and keep their patient functioning at the best possible level. What is offered by the clinic, or a health system, or social services, or local and voluntary organisations, varies all over the world.

What they could offer will be either pharmacological or non-pharmacological.

◆ Pharmacological – that is, drugs. In terms of medicines there are two pathways. If you've been diagnosed with Alzheimer's disease there are some drugs that can be offered. The drugs available are called cholinesterase inhibitors.

These drugs work something like the 'house that Jack built': i.e. 'this is the dog that barked at the cat that ran after the mouse', or here 'these are the drugs that inhibit the proteins that break down the chemicals that are important for memory'. They therefore have the effect of increasing acetylcholine, the brain's major 'memory chemical'. (Professor Kenneth Rockwood, Dalhousie University)

◆ Non-pharmacological – that is, support and advice on lifestyle changes and everything else.

The person might also be offered support for psychological problems such as depression and anxiety, both of which are understandable in the circumstances, and this could be either medicines or some behaviour therapies. Everyone should be offered post-diagnostic support.

In addition the clinic can offer support for other symptoms, which are called 'non-cognitive' or 'BPSD' (behavioural and psychological symptoms of dementia) and include hallucinations, delusions, anxiety, agitation and aggressive behaviour. Another expression that is used is 'behaviour that challenges' or 'disturbing behaviour' and this includes wandering, agitation, hoarding, sexual disinhibition, apathy and disruptive vocal activity (which basically means shouting out). Chapter 7 is devoted to disturbing behaviour and there it is made clear that much of such behaviour is an expression of distress.

We should assume the behaviour of a person has meaning even when we find it difficult to understand. What we might regard as difficult behaviour may in fact be a logical expression of fear, anger or frustration or the pain of the person with dementia. (Managing Disturbing Behaviour, dementia.stir.ac.uk)

The National Institute of Aging in the United States is quite clear about what should happen there.

A person with dementia should be under a doctor's care. The doctor might be a neurologist, family doctor, internist, geriatrician, or psychiatrist. He or she can treat the patient's physical and behavioural problems (such as aggression, agitation or wandering) and answer the many questions that the person or family may have.

People with dementia caused by Alzheimer's disease may be treated with medications. Four medications are approved by the US Food and Drug Administration to treat Alzheimer's. Donepezil (Aricept®), rivastigmine (Exelon®), and galantamine (Razadyne®) are used to treat mild to moderate Alzheimer's (donepezil has been approved to treat severe Alzheimer's as well). Memantine (Namenda®) is used to treat moderate to severe Alzheimer's. These drugs may help maintain thinking, memory and speaking skills, and may lessen certain behavioural problems for a few months to a few years in some people. However, they don't stop Alzheimer's disease from progressing. People with vascular dementia should take steps to prevent further strokes. These steps include controlling high blood pressure, monitoring and treating high blood cholesterol and diabetes, and not smoking.

What you can do

If you're concerned that you or someone you know has a serious memory problem, talk with your doctor. He or she may be able to diagnose the problem or refer you to a specialist in neurology or geriatric psychiatry. Healthcare professionals who specialise in Alzheimer's can recommend ways to manage the problem or suggest treatment or services that might help.

Participating in clinical trials is an effective way to help in the fight against Alzheimer's. To find out more about clinical trials, call the Alzheimer's Disease Education and Referral (ADEAR) Center toll-free at 1-800-438-4380 or visit the ADEAR Center website. More information is available at www.ClinicalTrials.gov. (http://www.nia.nih.gov/health/publication/forgetfulness)

What really happens?

We were the last appointment of the day. The doctor asked us to wait outside for a bit. Then he came out and told us that my wife had dementia. I went home in a complete daze. He gave us nothing ... not even a leaflet. We couldn't speak to each other. We didn't know what to say. (Couple in their 70s)

People with dementia can miss out on getting a diagnosis by a proper pathway. Your doctor might be one of those who don't recognise the value of a diagnosis. Your local memory assessment service may be so busy that the doctor does not bother to refer you because he thinks you will wait too long and achieve nothing of value.

We were trying to convince the doctors at their group practice meeting to make more diagnoses. I pointed out that this health centre ought to have forty or fifty more people on their register according to the statistics for the local older population. I even reminded them that they would get money from the government for doing it through something called QOF [quality and outcomes framework] points. One young doctor got really incensed. 'Even for money I will not do this,' he said indignantly. 'There is no benefit to my patient in going through these tests. There's no treatment for them.' Sir Galahad, it turned out, had no idea about the twenty-four-hour helpline, the befriending service, the financial support from the local authority and, to be honest, the human right of the patient to access information about themselves. For him 'treatment' means 'prescriptions'.
(English dementia diagnosis project leader)

It might be that you get a second chance of being given a diagnosis if you have to go to hospital for something else. All hospitals in the UK are supposed to check you for cognitive problems when you are admitted, particularly if you are older and appear confused. In some cases, although the check is done and the staff 'know' you've got dementia, it does not get written in your discharge letter so your doctor does not 'know' and neither the doctor nor the hospital refers your case to the memory assessment service. That's not good.

The person with dementia may be in a care home before someone actually puts a name to the problem.

Our mom was living at home by herself and me and my sister were taking good care of her. My sister works days in an office and I'm a delivery driver on nights, so we could always drop in at different times – shopping, doing chores, just a coffee. She had a fall and she was in hospital. We wanted her home. When she did get back they said she had to go to a clinic. We never knew what it was about because we just took her there and waited for her. It was called Outpatients B. She went back and forward a few times. Then she had another fall and broke her hip. We all decided she'd be better in a care facility, and she went to one to try it out and they said they couldn't have her because she had 'dementia'. No one had ever told us that for the two years we'd been taking her back and forward. If I'd have known maybe I could have done more and stopped her falling. No one told us what to do. No one told us nothing. (Son, aged 56, of his 75-year-old mother)

Of course, the process of getting a diagnosis is not always bad, but knowing some of the pitfalls will help you negotiate the symptoms.

I was very confused and anxious and my doctor really listened to me. Of course when I got to the memory clinic and it turned out to be dementia I was devastated, but I can't fault the wonderful staff who have supported me every step of the way. I want them to know now how grateful

I am that they are there for me. I'm determined to stay
well for as long as possible. My friends are all around me,
including the nurses and doctors. (Enid, 65)

And what if you don't have dementia ...

Well, that is a reason to be cheerful, surely, as long as
you and your doctor have got to the bottom of whatever
was making you worried. Get that infection treated, or
sort that vitamin problem, or deal with that stress and
get out of there!

It might be that they've decided you have mild
cognitive impairment, which generally affects older
people and means that, although you can function very
well, your mental strength is declining faster than in the
majority of people. One major difference from 'real'
dementia is that in about half of the people affected
it never gets really bad or descends into dementia. Of
course it is a nuisance, but if you follow the advice in
this book about keeping well, and even use some of the
techniques and technology described here, you'll still
be able to get on with your life as you wish and perhaps
reverse those symptoms.

To stay well with MCI you may decide to adopt the
same lifestyle changes that are known to help delay
symptoms in people who really do have dementia. You
want to keep your brain in the best shape possible, so
think about the following:

◆ Keep up all your normal activities as much as you can
for as long as you can.

◆ Keep your mind active. There is no single preferred activity, so the one that you enjoy most will be the best because you are more likely to stick at it.

◆ Keep involved with family and friends and enjoy community life through your usual activities, like going to church or meeting friends in the pub … whatever is usual for you.

◆ Plan ahead for situations that might become tricky, like dealing with banks and insurance (this includes arranging a power of attorney now, while you are well, for someone you trust to take care of decisions if the time should come when you are not up to it: see Chapter 13 for advice on legal issues).

◆ Get your medications checked regularly. The rule of thumb is that if you are on more than four it's possible that you are taking too many. The pharmacist can help check this out for you.

◆ Keep an eye on your blood pressure and cholesterol levels. Diet is really important for you now.

◆ Exercise, exercise, exercise … This is so important. You don't have to power round the gym, just make sure you keep moving.

◆ Stop smoking. Now. Immediately. No arguments. If your brain is struggling it needs more fuel. The fuel it likes is oxygen. Would you put the wrong fuel in your car knowing that it would be fatally damaging? You don't want to write off your brain, do you?

◆ The story is similar with alcohol. You need to preserve brain cells, not destroy them. The good news is that a glass of wine a day is a good thing. But if one is never enough for you it is better to have none at all.

◆ Reduce stress however you can and get enough sleep.

Is it impolite to suggest someone has dementia?

Because I'm known as a dementia expert, people are always asking me about dementia. Even at family gatherings or parties, people will come up and say, 'Do you think I've got it?' or 'Will I get it?' I find this openness hard to match with the reluctance that people have to raise such questions with each other. I've promised my own family that if they do show signs I'll tell them. This is because the medicine works best at the early phases and I don't want them to miss out. But I know that others do not raise the matter with relatives because it might seem insulting or frightening to suggest that they appear to be failing in some way.

If you are worried about being too direct, you could try supporting a local Alzheimer's charity fundraiser and going together to the part where they do a little talk about facts and figures. That will help you to open the conversation, especially if they are giving the message that earlier is better for diagnosis. Talk about your own fears and worries about the possibility of having dementia and describe what you'd do if you ever thought you had it, and then ask them what they'd do.

It might be that you just have to take the bull by the horns. You can appeal to the desire that many older people have not to be a nuisance. With my own parents

I made it clear that it is easier for everyone else if you get it checked out sooner rather than later. Their own altruism would be repaid because it is also usually better for the person with dementia. Overcome the stigma and taboo that you carry inside. Do your homework and make sure that you yourself see signs that are more than normal forgetting. Then be strong, as you would with any friend or family member at risk.

I said to her, 'Mother, there is so much about dementia in the news and I'm terrified that you might get it but miss out on all the medication and other help, so you MUST come with me and see about it. I insist. I'll come with you. If you are OK that's fine, but if not you'll cause us so much trouble later if you don't help us by dealing with it now. And it's not about you being forgetful, because we all have that. I just want to be sure you get tested.' (Daughter of Shakira, 79)

If the process during which the doctors ask the questions is annoying, be as supportive as you can. Most of what doctors have ever done to us is annoying, but we put up with it because they are wonderful and save our lives, or at least make them better. At this stage of life we can't do much about the stigma of 'failing' an exam, so until the doctors get more subtle in their testing techniques, make for home straight afterwards and be comforted in any way you can.

Getting a diagnosis of dementia can be a shattering experience. It is terrible luck, and everyone will be sad and upset for you. But then they must gather round you and make life the best it can possibly be … and this book will give you ideas for how that can be done.

chapter 3

Adjusting to the news: for caregivers

I've learned that people will forget what you said, people will forget what you did, but people never forget how you made them feel. (Maya Angelou)

When someone close to you is diagnosed with dementia the effect can be devastating. It is the responsibility of the doctor to tell the patient, and it should be done face to face at a special appointment so that the patient can ask questions. They should have someone with them and this may be you. This is a pivotal day in your lives. It is important to get as many facts as possible, so try to take notes or ask for some written information. If the doctor is not using language you understand, interrupt them to ask questions. They might use jargon or technical terms and it is essential to ask about what they mean – they won't mind. The doctor might not try to cover every stage of the illness in the first meeting, but you should not leave without some idea of what the next step is. If you arrive home and discover that you missed the next step, you can get back in touch and ask when the time is right for you.

Remember that technically the doctor must have the consent of the person with dementia before imparting personal information to you, the caregiver. That consent is implied by the person taking you to the consultation, so there should be no difficulty in you taking part in the conversation. Sometimes doctors are overly cautious about confidentiality, so be prepared to make a case. In Scotland, for example, caregivers' rights to be part of these conversations are enshrined in law. If the person you care for can't make a decision about their health care without your help, you should be involved in decisions. You have the right to ask for a second opinion from another doctor if you are unhappy with the decision that the health professional has made. In other places, caregivers always need to have a power of attorney (see Chapter 13) before they are allowed to be so involved.

Of course it is bad news that someone has such a serious condition, but there is an increasing awareness that the actual process of breaking the news will seriously affect how the person is going to live from then on. This can mean different things to different people. You and the patient might be pleased to have a name to put to what is wrong.

I thought I was going mad. I thought people were breaking into my house and stealing money. Now I know it is dementia, I'm not happy about it but it is less frightening. (Retired government official, 78)

The information that is being given may adversely affect the person's view of their future, with the prospect of limited choices and threats to their dignity and independence. In some cases, when done well, it can actually start a positive process of living well and extracting the best from the rest of life. Reluctance to give bad news has always been an issue in health care and doctors in the past have felt they had the right to withhold information. Doctors used to avoid telling people that they had cancer, even when it was clear that this must be the case because of the obvious treatments. What else do you get radiotherapy for? Sometimes they even withheld this information at the request of families.

Dad told me that Uncle Bill didn't want Aunt Sarah to know she had cancer. I was a young nurse at the time and I thought it was awful. We all knew, why not her? So I worked out a way of being alone with her and asked her if she wanted me to talk about her treatment. She gave me a smile and said, 'It's all right, darling. I know all I need to know.' There they were keeping their secrets and I know she knew perfectly well. It was them that needed to avoid facing it, not her. (Nurse)

It has been made clear to professionals in their guidelines that they must respect the right of the patient to know any bad news, while using professional judgement about how and when to give the full picture. Dementia care will remain far behind in achieving this standard while we still have clinicians who can't or won't address the issues.

What can you do to help?

Just by being there you have made a very good start. Not everyone has someone who cares about them at this time. You will feel anxious and devastated yourself and that needs to be dealt with, but later. This is not about you. If you are not able to be calm, you'll not be in a position to help.

When the doctor told us that Mom had dementia our world seemed to fall apart. She was so young. It was so unfair. But I had to be strong for her. I knew that the first couple of days would be the worst. She needed more information so that she could start to plan for the future. (Daughter of Ethel, 61)

When you come out of the consultation just calmly say what you are going to do next.

I got her in the car and drove her along to the abbey, and we sat on a bench near the lake. We've been there hundreds of times and I know she loves it. I had a flask of coffee with me. I must have known we were going to need it. We hardly spoke. (Husband of Ethel, 61)

You can't assume that you know what is most devastating about the news for the person concerned. It might be that her worst pain is the knowledge that she won't see her grandchildren get married, or that she's not going to be able to retire to the coast as she always planned. Don't try to hurry anything. This dementia thing can go on for years and this is just the first day. She may have years of good health ahead of her, but this is not the time to talk about that. You are both reeling from a blow. At some point you will have to think about how and when you are going to tell other people about it all, but perhaps not yet.

Right now you are filled with care and compassion for

the other person, but it's important not to be a hero. You may have to bear the brunt of anger and grief, in addition to dealing with the problems that have arisen as a result of the illness, which might include questions about future finances, car driving and how to just live together. So you need to find out how to care for yourself.

Everyone responds to these challenges in different ways. I am in awe of the caregivers I meet and how they manage. Here are some of the negative aspects of caring, with ideas on how to deal with them if you are affected.

Denial is a coping mechanism. It gives you time to adjust, but you can't stay like that for ever. At some point the caregiver has to start looking at the practical implications of what is happening and get the information that is needed to work out a plan for the future. But that doesn't happen in the first stage.

Anger is understandable. Your frustration and concern about how unfair this is may build up so much that you want to express them, but you need to find a place where it is safe to do so. In the heat of the moment it is possible to say things that you will later regret. You may have worked hard all your life, looking forward to a leisurely retirement, which now looks like being stolen. Of course you are angry.

Grief will arise from the sorrow you feel for what the other person is losing, and what you are losing yourself. To begin with you will have difficulty in thinking about anything else. You may lose yourself in sleep and then wake the next morning to feel it flooding in again. You need rest and distraction from it. This intense feeling, which is natural, will become less painful with time.

Thinking positively is a major challenge. Some of your negative thoughts are entirely rational, but you can focus on the problems too much. Live in the moment and try not to worry about the future or dwell on the past. Don't undervalue yourself and the wonderful work you are doing as a caregiver. Take consolation from your religion or faith. Take comfort from friends and family.

Resilience is the ability to recover from setbacks. You still feel the anger, grief and pain, but you can keep functioning. To do this you need to take care of yourself and not be afraid to ask others to help take care of you. Your resilience may be knocked, but you can recover.

Social isolation does happen when dementia strikes. It is really important to understand that friends are not a luxury; they are a necessity for maintaining your health and sanity. You need friends in order to be happy and you may need to tell them overtly that you need them. If you give them specific jobs to do for you it will help them know what you need from them.

Anxiety about the future is a common problem for care-givers at the time of diagnosis. The best antidote to this is to get as much information as you can about what support is available to you and what common problems you might face. You can get help and advice from a range of organisations listed at the end of this book.

Some caregivers do get affected by depression, exhaustion, sleeplessness, irritability and health problems, but many do not.

I joined the Alzheimer's carers association and it turned out they were looking for help with the accounts. That's my profession. My wife comes with me to the meetings, and she enjoys the company. We drop into the office two or three times a week and sometimes there are activities on that she can do while I'm toiling over the figures. A month ago we went to the legislature to a meeting to tell elected representatives about the needs of people with dementia. I feel a new lease of life. I didn't know about dementia before, but now I do I am determined to make the situation better for those coming after than they were for us. (John, retired accountant, 72)

Caregivers around the world

In some languages there is not even a word for 'carer' or 'caregiver' because in those cultures caring for someone when they are sick and vulnerable is simply what you do. People use the word 'carer' in the UK because the systems need to identify the people who are doing the work of caring. There are 'carer's allowances' and 'carer's assessments' and 'carer support groups'. You can't access any of these unless you are identified as a carer or caregiver.

Organisations like Carers UK are there to help people in Great Britain and Northern Ireland with advice on caring – but also with companionship at what can be a lonely time. Their details are at the end of this book. In Scotland there is a website called Care Information (www.careinfoscotland.co.uk/home.aspx) and NHS Choices in England has a wealth of wide-ranging information for carers on their website (www.nhs.uk/CarersDirect/yourself/Pages/Yourownwellbeinghome.aspx). This includes advice on getting time off work, types of caregiver breaks, how to take care of yourself, managing relationships and other issues, including hints for male caregivers who sometimes face practical problems because our society in general sometimes expects caregivers to be female, which is wrong. This advice is backed up by tools to assess your physical fitness and mental well-being. They take only moments to use and are connected to good advice about staying well. You have to look after yourself if you are going to be able to help others.

The American organisation The National Alliance for Caregiving (www.caregiving.org) serves as the Secretariat for the International Alliance of Carer Organizations, a coalition dedicated to recognizing the issues facing carers across the globe including members from Canada, Ireland, Australia, New Zealand, Sweden, the UK, the USA and Finland. Through these organisations and their websites a great deal of useful information is available. They may be able to help you to find who is near you and can help you in your task.

The American Society on Aging has created a list of twenty-five organisations that take care of caregivers. (www.asaging.org/blog/25-organizations-take-care-caregivers). One example is the AARP Caregiving Resource Center which provides family caregivers with information, tools and resources to help them. The site provides access to caregiving experts in various areas who provide information and a method of contacting other affected families.

At the end of this book is information about other societies and organisations that might help.

Check what services your local Alzheimer's Society may provide including:

◆ *individual and family support*

◆ *support groups for caregivers*

◆ *MedicAlert® Safely Home® – a programme that helps identify the person with dementia who is lost and assist in a safe return home*

◆ *First Link® – an early intervention programme that gives people with dementia and their caregivers a direct connection to information and services in their community*

◆ *brain health activities*

◆ *education for health-care providers*

◆ *day programmes for people with dementia / respite care*

◆ *art and music therapy*

However, it is often the case that you have to undertake some research to find out what is available near you.

chapter 4

Adjusting to the news: for people with dementia

I felt totally alone, with the world receding from me in every direction, and you could have used my anger to weld steel. (Terry Pratchett, October 2008, describing when he was diagnosed)

To say I understand what happens to someone when they are told they have dementia would be to trivialise a catastrophe that I have not yet experienced. It is not for me to say. When first diagnosed, my friends with dementia tell me, it's hard to find anything positive to say or do. Dementia is a bad thing. The Alzheimer Europe website gives reflections from people with dementia about how it was when they were diagnosed:

We were diagnosed over two years ago but can still remember those first shattering feelings – shock, disbelief, fear, shame, feeling cut off … and feeling very alone. Your brain feels numb and you can't take it all in … But take heart, these first terrible feelings really do pass. We know – we've been there. (Pat, James and Ian, www.alzheimer-europe.org/Living-with-dementia/After-diagnosis-What-next/Diagnosis-of-dementia/Facing-the-diagnosis*)*

The NHS Choices England website says, 'Once the

initial feelings of shock have passed, it is time to move on and create an action plan for the future.' In a breath-taking list of what you should do, it mentions such elements as making a will and putting your papers in order. It's the shock of the mundane. It does not say, 'We are so, so sorry.' But it should say that, because of what we know the health system might be about to do to you.

It is a strange life when you 'come out'. People get embarrassed, lower their voices, get lost for words … It seems that when you have cancer you are a brave battler against the disease, but when you have Alzheimer's you are an old fart. That's how people see you. It makes you feel quite alone. (Terry Pratchett, discussing stigma in dementia)

People with dementia are often very angry, because in addition to the unfairness of the disease they are dismayed by the exclusion they experience, even when people are talking about dementia and about them.

It may be hard for people with dementia to speak out, but Hilary Doxford has her words to the 2013 G8 Dementia Summit in London England preserved for all to see:

I feel fear and dread of what is to come, in particular of the day I no longer recognise Peter, my husband. I feel my quality of life will be on a steep decline from that point and I will be at the mercy of others …

I feel despair that, having received a diagnosis of dementia, there is no cure – just a long slide towards

*oblivion. As things currently stand, any cure will probably
be too late for me and the thousands like me …*

*I do have some hope – hope for the research that is in
progress, that it may deliver just in time for many of us, at
least to buy us more time. I hope that the funding can be
found to dramatically increase research work into finding a
cure, because the cost will be repaid so many times, not only
economically but also in the quality of life and happiness for
those affected (both patients and carers) …*

*I hope that I can live my life to the full and not just
exist. I hope that I have time to create more happy memories
for my husband to help him through dark times. (Hilary
Doxford, 54, describing her feelings on being diagnosed,*
www.dementiachallenge.dh.gov.uk)

Alzheimer Europe brought together people with
dementia to talk about what it means for them. Their
words are in a manual entitled *Alzheimer's Disease: After
the Diagnosis – What Next?* Dr James McKillop, MBE,
who himself has a diagnosis of dementia, was instru-
mental in reviewing drafts of that manual (and this
book) to make sure that the information is relevant and
understandable. The message is clear. Dementia does
not define people, though their powers will be limited
in a range of ways over time. I am inspired by my friends
with dementia who just keep going:

*… if we don't do it – who will? The stigma-filled conference
organisers who honestly believe we have no interest/
drive in helping ourselves, each other, and in educating
people like them? (Dr Richard Taylor, Dementia Alliance
International, who lived with dementia, responding to an*

online discussion about dementia events that marginalise
people with dementia. Dr Taylor died of cancer in 2015,
and remains an inspiration to people with dementia and
those who work with them.)

Sometimes angry people get organised and take collective action. James McKillop was one of the founder members of the Scottish Dementia Working Group, a politically active forum made up of people with dementia in the north of the UK. When undertaking a one-year project called DEEP (the Dementia Engagement and Empowerment Project) in 2012, the Joseph Rowntree Foundation discovered that there were not many groups led by or actively involving people with dementia that were influencing services and policies in England. Being involved at the time when you are just coming to terms with a diagnosis can be difficult. Campaigning and activism are different from being in a support group, but those involved often say that the support from an action group and the sense of empowerment are really significant when other supports are fading away and power seems to have been stripped away from you. The friendship and camaraderie are important. Time, fatigue and cost have all been identified as barriers to involvement. At the Alzheimer Europe conference in Malta in 2013 a Czech woman with dementia, Nina Baláčková, spoke of her personal experience of dementia and what it was like being part of the European Working Group of People with Dementia. There was standing room only for her speech, and the place was filled with people with dementia, caregivers, care workers and researchers who were inspired and moved by the discussion. She said, 'You can't choose what you feel, but you can choose what you do with it.'

Other people with dementia are emphatic about the importance of living well:

There is much research going on all over the world, which, I think and pray, one day will lead to prevention and/or a cure. But it is some way off. Until then make sure the person makes the most of their life. While there are drawbacks, I still enjoy living. I meet so many interesting people I would never have met did I not have dementia. I bask in their genuine friendship. I do miss a regular wage and driving, but hey, people in graveyards would gladly change places with me. I savour the life I currently have. (James McKillop)

Anyone who wonders what it feels like to have dementia should look at the on line forums for people who have dementia, where contributors talk to each other about how their day-to-day life is. In response to a man newly diagnosed with dementia, a registered user says:

Greetings ... I won't say welcome because this is a place that you probably don't want to be. Please know that this is a place where you can share what's going on with you, you can get a lot of loving support, and find comfort from those who know what you're feeling. You can look back on my posts, and see my story, but I was diagnosed at 54 years old with dementia, and I'm three years in.

A couple of things that work for me:

◆ *people diagnosed with dementia presents itself differently ...*

No two are the same

◆ *everybody is on different medications and every medication doesn't work the same on each person*

◆ *this is a road that nobody chooses to go down, but the more educated you are on what's happening, the more accepting you are of what's going on, the less frustrating*

◆ *try to take each moment, each day, as it comes.*

Lots of hugs and blessing coming your way.
(www.alzheimers.org.uk online forum, 1 February 2014)

In aircraft safety announcements you are told to put on your own oxygen mask before assisting other people. On ferries you are told to put on your own life jacket first. Remember to take care of yourself, otherwise you won't be able to help support others or participate in raising awareness and getting real political action on dementia. Tell other people that they must help you, and if they don't know how, recommend some of the later chapters in this book.

chapter 5

What are friends for?

A friend is someone who knows the song in your heart and can sing it back to you when you have forgotten the words.

Dementia presents a particular problem to friends if you are not part of the family. You might not know much about it yourself and the whole idea of it is terrifying. You want to help, but you are afraid of being embarrassing or inappropriate and you just don't know what would make a difference. Reading this chapter will provide guidance on what often does make a difference, based on what people with dementia and their family caregivers say.

We often get advised to 'keep up with friends'. This is the first time I've seen advice for friends to help. It is so badly needed, why has it not been done before? The Government and local authorities will have to take notice as it can save them a lot of care costs. (James McKillop)

Simple and easy-to-implement ideas for helping and staying with a friend through this dark time are presented here, together with potentially tricky scenarios, and also illustrations of how to cope and hints for how to have a conversation and be with people who have dementia.

Treat us as normal people. We're still here, just a little slower and sometimes confused.

This quote is from the Alzheimer's Disease International *World Alzheimer's Report* 2012, which focused on the times and the places where awkwardness, humiliation and shame are associated with dementia. The report brings to light some important views from family caregivers of people with dementia who if they were writing this would say:

◆ I do want and need help.

◆ I spend more time on caring than you think.

◆ I am isolated by my twenty-four-hour responsibility.

◆ I am judged by the rest of my family for the quality of my caring.

◆ I may not take the initiative in keeping up with our relationship.

◆ I may not be able to afford some of the support that is available.

◆ I have health and stress problems because I am a carer.

If people with dementia who were interviewed for the report were writing this they would say:

◆ I am aware that you are afraid to talk to me.

◆ I would like to be included in conversations.

◆ I would encourage you to ask me about whether I

want to discuss memory loss, because I might often want to.

◆ I know my own limitations.

◆ I want you to ask me if I want you to help me remember words I forget.

◆ I would often prefer you not to correct what I say, but show me you understand the meaning.

◆ I am disheartened when you avoid or ignore me.

◆ I am humiliated when you talk to my relative and not to me.

◆ I don't want to be a burden, so I hold myself back from things I'd like to do with you.

◆ I won't be taking the initiative as much any more.

As a friend who wants to help, you can do no better than respond to what the caregivers and people with dementia say.

What the carers would say

I do want and need help

If you want to help, it's really important to ask what would be most helpful. It might not be what you imagine. You might think getting in some food would be good, when in fact going to the market is the one outing the caregiver has to look forward to. Maybe they'd rather have transport to the mall or market, or they'd rather that you stay in their home with the person with dementia while they go out shopping on their own.

Some people find it very hard to accept help even though they need it. It may take time for them to work out what they are comfortable with asking for.

I say to caregivers, 'When you have time, sit and make a list of all the things that would help you, and when someone asks, show them the list and see if there is anything on there that they feel they can do.' If you've always been independent, or the person who gave help, it can be hard to reverse that position. (support worker)

You will see in Chapter 6 that one of the most important things for staying well for a person with dementia is exercise. Just think, if you offer to take them for a walk when you are taking your dog out (or push them in a wheelchair if they are beyond walking), you can get four times the benefit. Dog enjoys walk, person with dementia gets health benefits, caregiver gets an hour of respite and you get exercise! What's not to love about that? You might even help them sleep that night, which makes five benefits. It is the gift that keeps giving.

Doing activities with the person with dementia supports the caregiver with their burden. 'Burden' is such an awful word, because it sounds like something you'd want to put down. The caregiver does not always want to put it down.

I'm not her 'caregiver'. She's my wife. After fifty-five years I could not sleep without her in the bed beside me. Why would I want her to be in a home? (Frederick, 79)

There is no end to the list of useful chores you can do, including help with the garden, doing care and repair jobs, help with forms and correspondence, transport to church, taking round a cooked meal once a week, putting out the bin for the refuse collection, lending the latest DVD movie – being a friend in need. Not being sexist, but there are plenty of 'man' jobs and 'woman' jobs and you can make up for the gender imbalance in their house. If the man with dementia used to deal with clearing up the yard, be a hero and do it for him. In some countries, older couples may have been in the habit of leaving the driving to the husband, so be sensitive and try to help if one of them is not used to driving. In other places older men have not been used to cooking or other domestic tasks. It is hard to expect him to learn that on top of all the other challenges he may be facing. Even if you can't cook for him, you can do other things to leave him free to tackle his challenges.

Michael our neighbour is a firefighter. Without any comment he just mows our lawn when he's doing his own. He just invited himself in one day and checked out all the smoke detectors and replaced the batteries. It's hard to know how I can repay him and his family for their kindness, but they let us look after their dog once in a while when they are out. (John)

I spend more time on caring than you think

The best of our good friends have no idea how much time this takes up. If the caregiver goes out to work, they may spend hours there worrying, or making phone calls, or altering their work pattern to fit in with caring. Even if they have retired or had to give up their job, the caregiver may be woken up many times in the night and so is still exhausted. If you as a friend can give this person the gift of time, you will be doing the best you can. Time is rationed, and the caregiver does not have enough to guarantee their mental and physical health and personal safety. Donate time. You can do this either by house-sitting during the day, to let them get out, or at night, to let them sleep. You can undertake time-consuming tasks for them, using up some of your own free time. You can take the person with dementia away for long enough to give the caregiver a break. Encourage them to use the time for something that will really recharge their batteries. A play, a movie, a concert … these are nice highbrow activities. But to be honest some caregivers can't even use the bathroom without being interrupted, so don't be surprised if they seem not to have done what you'd think of as 'much' with the time. A shower, a shave and an uninterrupted visit to the toilet might be a real treat for a gentleman whose wife with dementia clings to him like a limpet, even following him to the bathroom.

I am isolated by my twenty-four-hour responsibility

Sometimes just being there and listening to the caregiver is helpful. If you take round some cakes, demand a cup of coffee and eat some together, just sharing time. You don't even have to go over if there is no time or your friend lives far away. There are excellent international examples of low-level support for isolated caregivers in the form of a regular phone call. Every morning the person gets a call from someone asking the usual things. How was your night? Are you doing anything today? How are you both? Did you see the news last night? Has this politician no shame? Why is the weather not as good as it was when we were young? Not many of us can survive for days without speaking to anyone other than the stranger who is emerging in our own home as dementia takes hold. A regular phone call can be a lifeline.

Not available regularly yourself or want to help someone you don't know? Check if your area has a resource similar to the UK's Silver Line Telephone Friend service:

What is a Silver Line Telephone Friend?
Silver Line Telephone Friends offer a befriending service, calling an older person once a week to check they are ok and to have a chat. We match older people to like-minded volunteers. All calls are free and managed using our 'virtual call centre' website. It is not a counselling service and Silver Line Friends will not ever meet or know the address of the people they speak to.

Please note for this role you will need

◆ *Access to the Internet*
◆ *A UK (or Channel Island or Isle of Man) landline telephone*
◆ *A commitment of approximately one hour per week for up to one year*

(http://www.thesilverline.org.uk/)

If you are searching for a non-profit social service organisation in your community try typing in the name of your city or state and the word 'aging' in your computer's browser. A number of organisations may show up, and you can ask them about caregiver support resources in your local area. You may find that one of them operates a telephone support service, based on the real experience of other caregivers, and professional or volunteer supporters.

It may be that the caregiver already has access to Skype or FaceTime and is familiar with electronic forms of communication, but if not you can help set them up. Of course they are not as good as being in the room with someone, but they open a window that people at the other side can use, like friends and family from far away. That window might be closed if you don't help the person to get online.

When you are inviting a caregiver to come out with you, or come to your house, make sure that they understand the person with dementia is welcome as well, and take care of both. I know that group meetings of caregivers might sound grim to you, if the people have nothing at all in common other than caring, but it can be incredibly useful. Help your friend to find and attend such a group if they want to.

I knew Alison had vascular dementia but it was only when someone said, 'Ask the Alzheimer's Society', that I realised they've got a meeting I can go to. I met a man just like me and his wife was the same as Alison. He did make me laugh. He says I made him feel better because he felt less alone. Now his wife has passed away he comes round sometimes and entices me out to a bar for a beer and to watch the football – not that I need much persuasion. (Frederick, 79)

I am judged by the rest of my family for the quality of my caring

Sometimes the judgement seems so unfair:

I've been going in to see my mother every day for two years, making her supper every night on the way home from work, before going home to cook for my family. Recently she got even more frail and it was taking longer and longer. I eventually had to get social services to get caregivers in to do the morning and evening for me on weekdays, and I go and do a big clear-up at the weekend and bathe and feed her then. Then I got this horrible phone call from my sister because she had called in and found strangers in the house. It's the first time she's visited in six months but she was horrible to me, calling me names and blaming me. (S.M., daughter)

The tension in families can be appalling, and if you are a friend you may have to listen to quite a lot of this. Hindsight is a wonderful thing and it might not help your relationship if you point out that it would have been a good idea to let the sister know about the change of circumstances. At least you now know the lie of the land, that the sister is unhelpfully oversensitive in one way and unhelpfully insensitive in another way, and if your friend is making any other changes you can prompt her to let the rest of the family know, galling though such a responsibility might seem to her.

I not only have to do it all, but I have to report back to the lazy witch as well! (S.M.)

Families who use social media can start a private blog, where everyone has their own responsibility to log in and find out for themselves what is going on. Keeping a diary of what is happening on top of everything else might seem a burden, but it has a number of benefits, including reminding everyone how much change has taken place. Check out the video about Grouple, which was a lively way for families to do this together (http://www.designcouncil.org.uk/resources/case-study/grouple). It never became commercially available, probably because WordPress and Blogger are widely available and can support private group blogs. Families could also use private Facebook groups. This is where the knowledge and strength of younger people comes to the fore. They know all about social media. Use their energy.

Families accuse each other of terrible crimes, and think that the caregiver is 'doing them out of' inheritance, or affection or things we can't even imagine. Of course if you thought the caregiver was abusing the person with dementia you'd inform the authorities. But if they are not and you are their friend, listen, listen and then listen some more. And find a way of sympathizing without throwing fuel on the fire. Two years from now the mother may be dead and those sisters will need to be the best support they can be for each other.

I may not take the initiative in keeping up with our relationship

If you invite someone a few times and they never take you up on the offer, the usual response is to take the hint and drop them. Once they have missed sending you a birthday or other greeting card a few times, you start to erase their name from your own list. You might just realise one day that you've not spoken for a year or two. Always, always be the one who makes the contact, if they are struggling with dementia in their family. The amount of time that they have is severely limited. Being with you might be a treat that they have denied themselves. The exhaustion from their tasks may give them the idea that they don't have time to wash and dress well enough to come out with you for a coffee, even if they could leave their loved one at home alone. Shame about the state their home is in might stop them, out of pride, from inviting you round.

If you are a friend you will know ways around this problem. Be patient and persistent and remember that this is not about you. Caregivers tell us that friends just stop calling and they are embarrassed to beg for attention. Socializing is one of the few activities that make a difference in dementia, so do it for the person with dementia if not for the caregiver. You can help both at once.

I may not be able to afford some of the support that is available

Even places where many services are free at the point

of use, have other services that would be useful but have to be paid for, even if they come through the local council. In many places the funding of care is complex. If you wonder why the person does not take up everything that is available, consider whether finance may be an issue. It is also possible that they just don't understand what is available.

Our home is worth a lot of money, I know, but there's not much cash now our investments are getting no returns. If I sell the house, she'll be even more confused by the move. We look rich but I can't afford the home help. I'm not having that means test. (Pat, 85, sister of Helen, 81)

For example, in the US there is a complex web of different financing arrangements. Medicare, the tax-based federal health insurance programme, is the main source of medical care for older people with dementia, whether that is in or out of hospital. Medicaid is the safety net for low income Americans, but the whole system is fragmented. The PPACA (Patient Protection and Affordable Care Act) includes provision for dementia care, but it will take time to implement this reform. More than half the cost is therefore still covered by families. There is huge variation between states and communities. It would be almost impossible, although that is one country, to advise on a way forward, so local knowledge is really important, and that can sometimes be got through Alzheimer organisations.

Many older people avoid social services and social work departments because they are afraid that they'll lose control of the situation. In the UK, as a friend you could do them a favour by making sure that they know about the 'wealth check' that can be done discreetly and privately by a charity like Age UK, through which they can find ways of maximizing their income they did not previously know about. A huge number of state allowances are never collected by caregivers. A family lawyer could help here, if they could afford the fee.

In addition to considering how to improve their finances, think of free or low-cost things that you can do together. If you invite them out for a meal they might say no because they can't pay or return the compliment if you pay. On the other hand, you could go for a walk in the park together, or attend the local farmer's market or shopping mall just to window shop even if you are not buying, or go with them to a place of worship ... or any other free activities that are available in your community. Remember that your company is what makes the difference, so find a way of providing that while preserving the dignity of the people affected.

I have health and stress problems because I am a carer

The research on stress and burden is extensive, but different people have different coping skills, so their profound commitment is not necessarily going to make them ill. Of the people who do get ill, they seem to have more health problems as the person with dementia gets more dementia problems. Most carer health problems can be reversed if they are given proper information and support. Just by being a good friend you can reduce the risk of this person having health and stress problems. You can help gather information and find out where there are other sources of support. And of course you can just be there for them.

Caregivers are a diverse bunch of people. They're not recruited against a job description and skills set. The timescale of their caring is relevant. In the run-up to getting a diagnosis there has been a worrying time for them and it can be a relief to know what was causing the problems. Conversely, the time when the person goes into a care home or nursing home, which some might think of as a relief, is a time of terrible loss and change, and constant worry about whether the home is doing the care properly.

The distinguished author Alan Bennett gives a moving account in *Untold Stories* of when his mother was taken into care. He talks about the 'casual cruelties that routine inflicts'. The staff washed her hair and left it 'so that it now stood out round her head in a mad halo, this straightaway drafting her into the ranks of the demented ... the change was so dramatic, the obliteration of her usual self so utter and complete, that to restore her even to an appearance of normality now seemed beyond hope. She was mad because she looked mad.'

In some families letting someone go into care is not considered as getting them the benefit of a skilled resource providing the best solution, but rather as a failure and a source of shame. Bennett talks about how neighbours learned not to ask about his mother. But friends can help with the transition, and you could take turns at visiting the home, or help the caregiver use their new-found free time to be a friend again in the old ways, going out and about. Remember that even when they are in a care or nursing home, the person with dementia can still be entertained by you, on or off the premises. That's another way of sharing the burden that has been borne by your friend.

What the people with dementia would say

I am aware that you are afraid to talk to me

To be honest, they've got more to be afraid of than you do. Imagine how it feels when someone vaguely familiar is coming towards you and you are searching for their name. It happens to all of us – at work, at a party, in the street. Your main concern is whether you are going to embarrass yourself.

You may be afraid of getting something wrong, but the person with dementia is at a stage in their life when they are getting lots and lots of things wrong, and remembering your face might just be another one of them. So save them from that. Walk up and introduce yourself. If you are really clever you can do it in a way that does not draw attention to the problem:

Doris and I were standing at the post office together and Ethel, who has dementia, came in. I said to Ethel when she got close to us, 'Hello, Ethel, how are you? Look, Doris, here is Ethel.' And Doris replied, 'How are you today? John and I were nearly late for church on Sunday.' I followed up by saying, 'Well, Ethel. You can tell everyone at the church that Doris and John are going to try to be on time.' We all laughed, and Ethel was nudged to remember that we are John and Doris she knows from the church. We don't usually use our own names much in conversation, but we make a point with Ethel, and we plant clues in what we say. If everyone did that she'd be able to join in more often. (Doris and John, friends of Ethel, 61)

As a busy professor in the dementia field, I meet thousands of people every year and I occasionally don't remember someone from a few months ago, or whom I met only briefly. The person I meet often assumes that I'll remember them better than I do, and it's embarrassing, because I don't want to insult anyone. That's a hazard of my job, and I find ways round it. However, a friend of someone with dementia would do their best to reduce the problems for them, so keep introducing yourself even when it seems a bit silly. Err on the right side.

I would like to be included in conversations

Remember what Maya Angelou said 'people never forget how you made them feel.'

To begin with there will be little change from what you are used to in your friend, but by the end the person may not have much language left. Dementia impairments are spread over a number of years, so the way of speaking with a person with dementia will change over time.

I myself find that I need things repeated as I did not hear them properly. I might have misheard a word which throws the whole sentence out. I usually turn to Maureen, who repeats the question and I can follow her voice. I am used to it. With some individuals I never know what they said and we always have to get Maureen to repeat for me. (James McKillop)

As the words disappear, non-verbal communication becomes more and more important. A hug, a handshake, linked arms or hands – all of these can communicate something right to the end. Smiles and just sitting together can be a great comfort.

However, if you want to converse, remember the following:

◆ The language difficulties will vary according to the type of dementia, but in general over time you need to leave more time for questions and comments to sink in, and for responses to come back.

We have been working with the telesales staff at the electricity supply company, and teaching them the 'ten second' rule – that's where you wait for ten seconds after asking a question before giving the person a prompt. You really need to give them time to answer. However it seems a very long time when you are hanging on the telephone, perhaps wondering if they heard or if they are still there on the end of the line. (SL, dementia teacher)

◆ Relax – it's the quality that counts, not the speed! (A great revelation for me was listening to a recording of a friend with dementia talking. When I played it at twice normal speed, he sounded coherent and fluent. When I had listened at normal speed, I wondered if he was making sense. My impatience with his speed of communication was making me judgmental about the content of what he was saying.)

◆ A person with frontotemporal dementia may start to say things that are a bit shocking or to use language that could be offensive. A friend will respond to what is good in what someone says, so don't respond to what you think of as bad. There is no point in starting an argument about whether they should curse. It's the illness cursing.

◆ Although it is important to keep your conversation at the right pace, and that is probably slower than your normal pace, avoid the risk of sounding like an infant school teacher talking to a child. It's not appreciated and it doesn't help. A friend must not treat you like a child, even if you have dementia.

◆ A person with dementia does not lose their sense of humour. My friends with dementia are among the funniest people I've been with. They flirt and tell vulgar jokes and are politically incorrect as much as the next person. Don't try to sanctify them.

◆ Here is a controversial point. I always say that if a person with dementia has not understood something, it's a good idea to say the same thing again. The Alzheimer's Society recommends you rephrase it. Maybe they are assuming that the friend said the first thing in a way that is too complicated and so needs to simplify it. Sometimes you do just need to say it again, and if you say it again differently, the person then wonders what they missed when you first spoke. You know the person, so just try what works.

◆ Listen very carefully and take time. I've found that even if the person sounds incoherent at first, when you stick with it the meaning does come out. It is like they are talking in 'Scribble'.

My grandmother used to behave as if she was chattering away, with mixed-up words, exclamations, nods and winks, and then a clear phrase would come through, out of context, like a clearing in fog that opened and closed again just as quick. We used to say she was talking in 'Scribble', a new sort of jumbled-up language which had real meaning to her. (J.M., granddaughter)

◆ Crowded places are difficult for chatting. Background noise makes attention really difficult in dementia, so don't try to have a big conversation in a crowded or busy place, and even in a domestic setting switch off the radio or TV in order to talk properly.

I would encourage you to ask me about whether I want to discuss memory loss, because I might often want to

As a friend of a person with dementia, you may well have read a bit about it. You are clearly reading this book anyway. So you probably want to know what kind of dementia it is, and what is likely to happen next. You might be afraid to ask because the answer might be distressing. We also have a natural reserve about personal questions. People are always talking about their own illnesses and their friends' illnesses, and keep gall stones in a jar on the bookshelf, but there is something intimate and potentially shameful about a 'mental' condition. If you are a friend you might be one of the few people that I can share my hopes and fears with. It might be that I want to talk to you about stuff I can't share with my family. At least let me know that you have an open door for that sort of conversation. And respect it if I say that my door is firmly closed. Things might change over time, though.

I know my own limitations

People sometimes wonder if the person with dementia is unaware of what is happening to them. More and more evidence is appearing that demonstrates they do know, and for much longer than we might think. In fact some people know that something is going wrong long before they can persuade a doctor or anyone else that they've got this problem. When you see the lengths to which people will go to conceal the impairments that are hitting them, it's clear that they know. The earlier the diagnosis, the more chance they have of finding out about the condition, what can be done to keep symptoms at bay and what the prognosis is.

The day after I got my diagnosis everybody started treating me like an idiot. (Arlene, 73)

As a friend, of course you will be worried about whether they'll get lost, or be swindled by people in stores, or let strangers into the apartment to rob them. But the person with dementia should be your guide as to what they can do. People with dementia are entitled to take risks and make unwise decisions – it's not up to their friends, and a good friend can support them in doing what they really want. You might have to help them stand up to others.

I want you to ask me if I want you to help me remember words I forget

The advice that is given when you are talking to a friend with dementia is not unlike the advice for talking to someone who has another communication disorder, like stuttering. Relax and take time. Don't raise your voice, because the problem is not deafness. Use normal eye contact: a hard stare would be really disconcerting, and you need to realise that your facial expression will be read and recognised by your friend, so be aware of it. Pay attention and show that you are listening with genuine interest and are not making judgements. If you interrupt and don't let them finish their turn at speaking it will be demoralizing. One problem in dementia is difficulty in finding words, and some people think it is really helpful if you offer the word. Consider that the person with dementia may find that depressing, because they believe that straining to find the word will make them better at finding other words – like a memory-strengthening exercise. If you are my friend and you 'find' the wrong word persistently you are going to be really annoying, so ask each person what they find most helpful and do what they want.

I would often prefer you not to correct what I say, but show me you understand the meaning

My gran used to talk to me in 'Scribble'. The words were all mixed up or made up. But if you looked in her eyes and listened to her tone you could tell what she was saying. 'Thank you for these beautiful flowers' ... or 'Where's Grandad, I really miss him' ... or 'I wonder who you are, but I think you're a kind girl' ... We could be together for hours like that. It reminded me of the 'concrete poems' they used to teach us at school in the Sixties. The intended effect of those was never in the literal meaning of the actual words used. (J.M., granddaughter)

Depending on the cause of the dementia, the words used by a person may start to seem unintelligible. When professionals sometimes say, 'She can't communicate,' they really mean, 'She can't communicate verbally in a way that I understand.' Verbal communication is not all it is cracked up to be. Ask any cat – they do fine without it. Remember that the person with dementia is more dependent than most people on non-verbal communication and still can read it, even if you can't. A sigh of exasperation or rolling of the eyes, which are unconscious movements on your part, will communicate themselves very clearly to the apparently 'uncommunicative' person before you. They'll read you like a book. Try to respond to your friend's version of 'Scribble'. Or get them a cat.

When your friend with dementia says no one ever comes to visit her, don't argue the fact that care workers come in three times a day, and the priest once a week, and the daughter every evening and you are standing there, living proof of visitors. Listen to the meaning underneath the words. What she is saying is that she feels abandoned and it does not matter at that moment that she's really not been abandoned. Work with what she feels and do something to distract her from that feeling for at least the time you are together. Talk about the past, show pictures, sing a song, or walk round the garden … just be together. Pray or meditate if that is what you would always have done. People with dementia get a really interesting emotional hangover in that if you upset them, they remain upset after they've forgotten what upset them. If you comfort and distract them happily, they remain happy long after they've forgotten your kindness and humour. You can help them to be happy even after you have gone.

I am disheartened when you avoid or ignore me

A friend would not stay away from a person with dementia. It is really helpful if you pay attention and offer companionship and kindness. Although this section is intended to be positive and practical, I know it is a tough gig being cheerful and friendly for someone who is losing their cognitive capacity and who might at some stage not even remember who you are. But you've got many options. If it is too hard to be with them for long and try to communicate, you can do something for their caregivers. People go out and support charities and walk the Great Wall of China to raise money in memory of people with dementia who were their friends. Somewhere, somehow, they will know that you are doing this and be grateful. Anyone can do that, but only a friend can take you for a game of golf, and not worry about the fact that you can't keep the score any more and sometimes face the wrong direction. A visit can make a difference, even though you might not think so at the time.

When I was in the Girl Scouts we had to do the 'visitor' badge test. It involved picking a solitary person we knew and going round to see them. I picked a retired schoolteacher who had previously taught me in elementary school. I was about sixteen. Looking back, I can see that she had dementia. She never knew I was coming even though it was all arranged. She would offer me tea and then not make it. She repeated the same things she'd said before. She'd even go out of the room and leave me alone and forget that I was in her house. Now I realise that what seemed like a futile box-ticking exercise for my badge was probably a really good thing. She was hard to visit, and as a result everyone else in her circle was ignoring her. I went six times and I wish now I'd kept it up. (Dementia nurse)

I am humiliated when you talk to my relative and not to me

The 'Does he take sugar?' cliché has entered our language as an expression for the syndrome where able-bodied people are unable to speak directly to a person with a disability. Friends may be embarrassed and even ashamed to catch the eye of the person with dementia. It is as if there might be something showing in their face, like pity or horror, which they don't want the person with dementia to see. You just have to get over that. Spend time, if you need it, talking about your horror with someone else, and prepare yourself to be with your friend without showing dismay. After all, this is their tragedy, not yours, and for once this is a tragedy with which you can help.

The person with dementia is often stripped of their dignity, even at the early stages of the condition, so you can be a role model for everyone else about how they should be supported and regarded properly. There is also a temptation for family themselves to start speaking for the person with dementia before this is remotely necessary. You can help with this by your example.

When someone with dementia makes jokes about dementia itself, the power base shifts. The potential for humiliation is reversed and people who are sanctimonious about dementia are put in their place. Fiona Phillips in the *Mirror* newspaper talks about Tony Booth, an actor who has dementia, and his contribution to a dementia meeting:

He walks in, a huge smile on his still-handsome face, accompanied by former teacher Stephanie, his fourth wife. His addictions now reduced to cigarettes and tea, he raises his cuppa and cheekily proclaims, 'I'll drink to that,' as the aims of the session are outlined. When the Alzheimer's Society volunteer asks the group, 'What do you think of when you see the word dementia?', always looking for a laugh, he shouts out, 'I've forgotten!' Later his eyes twinkle

as he asks, 'Is it true that men drive women demented?'
Much hilarity ensues ... (Mirror, 10 February 2014)

His ebullient personality intact at present, no one is going to talk to his wife about him in his presence. You need to be sure you don't do this accidentally to a less confident personality. It is worth noting that the jokes Tony Booth makes about dementia might be offensive if made by someone else. It is really bad manners to joke about dementia until you've got it. Then you can say what you like. I'm looking forward to that, in a way.

I don't want to be a burden, so I hold myself back from things I'd like to do with you

You may need to use strong encouragement to get the person to join in, because they have a fear of holding everyone back. They might want to join you on a trip abroad but be afraid to ask. They might want to climb one last mountain but feel that the responsibility for them is something you can't take on. They won't come to the club with you any more in case they embarrass themselves and you. As a friend you may influence the person with abundant demonstrations of attention and friendliness. Their self-esteem is low and their self-confidence even lower, so you will have to work hard to help them understand they are not a burden. The confidence of their friends will help make up for their own lack of confidence.

The strongest expression of this urge to avoid being a burden would be the inclination to commit suicide.

In that case the person with dementia is holding themselves back from even living. There is evidence that people with nightmare conditions such as motor neuron disease, faced with the horror of not being able to breathe or swallow, might consider suicide, or people with uncontrolled pain feel that they personally cannot bear to live with it. However, there is no evidence that people with dementia are actually more suicidal than other older people. But there are those who think they ought to be:

Elderly people suffering from dementia should consider ending their lives because they are a burden on the NHS and their families, according to the influential medical ethics expert Baroness Warnock. The veteran Government adviser said pensioners in mental decline are 'wasting people's lives' because of the care they require and should be allowed to opt for euthanasia even if they are not in pain ... Lady Warnock ... [is] a former headmistress who went on to become Britain's leading moral philosopher ... (Daily Telegraph, *London,18 September 2008*)

Sadly the data from the Netherlands indicates that people diagnosed with conditions like Alzheimer's disease are accepting euthanasia from doctors. The disturbing thing is that the rules on consent mean you have to undergo the fatal process before you have lost capacity, so the person dying has not experienced the thing of which they are afraid, but chose death to avoid it. A doctor is agreeing with them that dementia is worse than death. Everyone is different, but I worry that they are not afraid of dementia, but poor dementia care, or the burden and cost to their surviving family. I can think of nothing more tragic than the person who wishes to be killed because of the burden they are to other people. Other people have given them the view that they are a burden and friends can lessen that. So do everything you can to show that your friend with dementia is not a burden and have fun doing the things you both like as long as you can.

The idea is to die young as late as possible (Ashley Montagu, anthropologist)

I won't be taking the initiative as much any more

The final point is that you need to keep going even when you've reached the position where you are not sure that they know you. We do this out of humanity and our own self-respect, as much as for the benefit of our friends. This is what being human is. Being a friend right up till the end of life is the most precious gift in the world.

I felt privileged to be allowed to be involved and to help in looking after her a bit and supporting her husband. He's such a lovely man and he cared for her so beautifully. He deserved all the help and respect I could give him. (John, friend)

There are many practical tasks you can do to help, like undertaking simple chores, picking up prescriptions or fetching a newspaper. If you are the caregiver, don't hesitate to ask friends to help. But just being there is really important.

Piglet sidled up to Pooh from behind.

'Pooh?' he whispered.

'Yes, Piglet?'

'Nothing,' said Piglet, taking Pooh's hand. 'I just wanted to be sure of you.'

(A.A. Milne)

chapter 6

How to keep dementia at bay

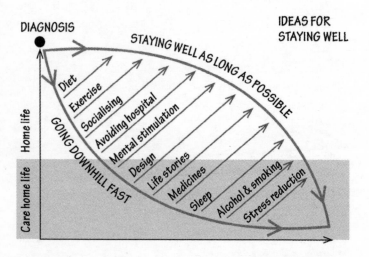

There are problems in providing evidence even for some of the more promising claims that are made about how to delay dementia. Research sometimes gives rise to apparently conflicting results. It is really challenging, for example, to design a research programme that tests the effect of one intervention and not another, such as only vitamins and not exercise, or only fish and not stress. As a result, studies appear to contradict each other, because the researchers were not measuring the same things, and they were not able to narrow their focus enough. Doing research on humans is complicated because we are complicated. This is especially true if you are measuring changes in behaviour, rather than easy to measure things like blood pressure, or pulse. Before listing here what is said to help, it is worth noting that this is your excuse to focus on the elements that you like best and can stick with. Take your pick, because most of it probably helps a bit. But if you are really interested in prevention and staying well, the thing for which there is the strongest evidence is exercise. That is one of the important messages in this chapter, though everything else described here will make some difference to someone, if not everyone.

The disease vs. the symptoms

The information available on the Internet and in newspapers is sometimes confusing because the journalist or reporter does not explain or perhaps even understand that there is a difference between 'Alzheimer's disease' (or Pick's disease, or vascular, or any other disease process – see Chapter 1) and 'dementia'. So when they highlight a new wonder food or activity that can 'slow Alzheimer's disease' they might be talking about slowing the rate of build-up of the plaques and tangles in the anatomy of the brain, or they might specifically be talking about slowing up one or other of the dementia symptoms. It is hard to follow the news when journalists use 'Alzheimer's' as a synonym for any 'dementia', no matter what the cause, and when they don't distinguish between the different symptoms, like memory loss, difficulty in working things out, stress reactions, or difficulty in learning new things. And sometimes the experiment turns out to have been so far only on mice, which is encouraging. But it is frankly misleading when the headline implies that it's about humans.

In considering why there are so many misleading headlines, we have to look at how universities and research facilities work and are funded. These institutions are quite rightly dependent for their reputations on demonstrating impact from their work, and this means that their scientists are under pressure to report potential good news. Once this information is in the hands of public relations specialists and the popular press, it gets reworded and simplified until it is so changed as to be possibly misleading. No one is being accused of lying, just wishful thinking:

The news reporter asked me to comment on the research that had found a 'cure for dementia by electrical stimulation of the brain'. When I looked at the paper published by the scientists it was of some interest because they had made the brains of live middle-aged lab rats bigger by putting electricity through needles in their brains. However, it is a far cry from there to the idea that it might help humans with dementia. Those people are different because they are old, and not rats, and they have dementia-diseased brains. Human brains shrink in dementia but just plumping them up again does not necessarily 'mend' the bit that has been damaged. Nevertheless there will be people asking their doctor for this, and being bitterly disappointed. It might one day turn out to have been relevant, but reporting it in the paper today as a 'cure' is cruel. And even though I said this to the reporter, it still got printed. News values are not the same as health values. It's an entertainment industry, not an information industry. And we collude with that. (Dementia expert)

The most decisive medical measurement of the disease that caused the dementia unfortunately comes only from weighing and analyzing the brain tissue at autopsy. Because dementia symptoms are changes in how a person is behaving and thinking, you can observe those symptoms increase or decrease while the person is still alive. This measurement is done by clinicians and researchers using a wide range of tests. These experts choose which of the individual dementia symptoms, or which groups of symptoms are most relevant to their study, and use a test that measures those specific symptoms. The report in the newspaper may say that an intervention 'reduces Alzheimer's' when the research actually demonstrates only that it improves one particular symptom of dementia, such as memory. You can help with memory problems, one symptom of dementia, without reducing the Alzheimer's disease. And you can reduce one symptom of dementia, without affecting other symptoms of dementia. For example, in an experiment the memory might be better, but aggression and agitation might not have changed in a positive way. Pharmaceutical researchers are steered towards a particular interest in memory, but it might be that an intervention that fails to improve memory makes something else (something that is harder to measure) better:

This patient was tested to see if the medication was making any difference to her and the standard cognition tests were negative. Not enough improvement to make it worth the cost of the prescription. Then the family pointed out that since she got the medication she had started to play the piano again, having stopped doing that for a long time. From the research measurement point of view the medication was not working; but it transformed her in a way that mattered to her, and to the family. So can we say it did not work? (Abridged from a clinical report by Professor Kenneth Rockwood, Dalhousie University, Canada)

From a practical point of view we have to ask if it makes a difference to the patient whether you are slowing the underlying disease or slowing the symptoms. Personally, I do not care if my brain shrinks a bit as long as it is not too noticeable in my daily life. It's of no benefit to me if the medication stops the brain shrinking but my mental capacity continues to shrink. What matters to me most is the quality of my daily life. That may be improved or maintained to a certain extent even while the pathology is taking greater hold.

It is as if we are saying here that some things work which we are told don't work, and some don't work which we are told do. How hard is it to make sense of all of this?

There are some interventions that may affect the underlying diseases and there are some interventions that affect only the symptoms. For example, later in this book (page 215) you will find advice on increasing light levels in the place where you live. That does not affect the rate at which the brain shrinks, but it does reduce the level of dementia symptoms experienced by the person. It would be good to try to do both, but while the scientists are struggling with the former, you can still roll up your sleeves and get on with the latter. There is something practical that you can do.

So the recommendation is this: the things that you can do that we think might keep dementia at bay are worth sticking with (or starting) even if you already have a diagnosis. They will help you to stay well, and so keeping them up as long as possible is a really good idea.

Drugs

I will do anything in my power to help them find a medicine for dementia, even if it is too late for me. (Volunteer with dementia in the Scottish Dementia Clinical Network cohort)

◆ There is at present no medicine that will prevent the development of the underlying diseases that cause dementia, except those medicines that will help with depression, blood pressure management, cholesterol management, diabetes, and the like. If you have any of those diseases your treatment for them and management of them are important, because all of them predispose a person to developing dementia.

◆ Everyone is looking very hard for a drug or vaccine to prevent dementia, because apart from the humanitarian issues, the financial rewards of such a discovery would be amazing. This is why you might get upset when people complain that they have found a 'cure' and no one is listening to them. Believe me, if there was anything in it, they'd be better keeping quiet until they get the patents sorted out. We all want that cure and it's worth a fortune. Just shortening the disease process by a year could save 10 per cent of the total cost, which would be enough money to build a lot of hospitals and care homes.

◆ The medication that is currently licensed for use around the world is mainly for the Alzheimer's form of dementia and is usually prescribed in the early and middle stages of the disease, when the maximum benefit is derived from them. This is a primary reason why early diagnosis is seen to be a good idea by doctors and this has helped to get an increase in access to diagnosis. The aim of the medication is to stabilise the condition. Not everybody will benefit from these drugs. They have side effects, including nausea and vomiting, and they can lower the pulse rate unhelpfully. It is often said that they only delay the progress of symptoms, but they also appear to have an impact on the pathology that underlies the diseases that cause the symptoms. Either way, they are all we've got in the medicine cabinet. The medications for use in different countries have in some cases different brand names. Cholinesterase inhibitors have names like donepezil (Aricept®), rivastigmine (Exelon®), galantamine (Razadyne®).

◆ These medications work by boosting levels of
a chemical messenger involved in memory and
judgement. Side effects can include nausea, vomiting
and diarrhea. Although primarily used to treat
Alzheimer's disease, these medications may also treat
vascular dementia, Parkinson's disease, dementia and
Lewy body dementia. Another medicine, memantine
(Namenda®) works by regulating the activity of
glutamate. Glutamate is another chemical messenger
involved in brain functions, such as learning and
memory. A common side effect of memantine is
dizziness. Some research has shown that combining
memantine with a cholinesterase inhibitor may have
beneficial results.

Smoking and alcohol

*The gentlemen who live here now have had difficult
lives. Their families and former friends, often because of
behaviours in the past that were a result of use of alcohol,
reject them. We do not ask questions or judge them. Some
of them cannot remember what happened three minutes ago
but will tell you in great detail about a drinking party they
had on their eighteenth birthday. The degradation of their
faculties and what they have lost is tragic. Their limited
lives are in sharp contrast with the macho culture which
gave rise to their disabilities … [In response to a question]
Yes, many of them have military backgrounds and had
distinguished service careers in theatres of war. (Matron of
care home)*

◆ Alcohol-related brain damage (ARBD) is the only

preventable form of dementia. Women's brains are more vulnerable to alcohol and women who drink 'in moderation' have an increased risk of mild cognitive impairment. People who indulge in binge drinking, such as having a heavy session once a month, are more likely to experience problems, and fortnightly bingeing doubles the risk. People of all ages need to take care, but drinking in older age presents its own problems.

◆ Research into the use of alcohol by people in different ethnic communities is limited. What people say is sometimes inaccurate and a generalisation. There are different patterns of use, but this can be because of historical and cultural factors, not genetics or physical differences other than size and sex. However, there are some ethnic differences in the rate at which people process alcohol in their bodies. The longer it is circulating before it is processed and excreted, the more dangerous it is for your brain. For example, Native Americans appear to metabolise alcohol more slowly.

There is research that shows having one glass of red wine a day can have beneficial effects. I prefer champagne. Fortunately, recent research from the University of Reading suggests that people over forty would be wise to drink two or three glasses of bubbly a week. Hurrah! That research was done with rats, but I don't care. In this case, because I like champagne, it's good enough evidence for me. (I'm only saying this to highlight that people demonstrate a lot of personal bias in what they are prepared to believe.)

◆ Don't smoke. It would be better if you never had, but improvements will start the day you give up. There is clear evidence of this in the case of heavy smokers. If you give up in middle age, the risk of dementia after twenty years is the same as if you had never smoked. There is an obvious link with vascular health, but it is linked to risk of Alzheimer's disease as well.

◆ If the management of drinking and smoking is challenging for you, remember that there are helplines and organisations there to support you. You can contact these through your doctor, or search the Internet for local support groups. In countries like the United States, Canada and Australia, those health-harming habits may be more prevalent in minority ethnic communities and specific services are focused on them.

Here is an example of a programme from Australia:

Quit Victoria has a number of strategies to reach culturally and linguistically diverse (CALD) communities including:

◆ ***Resources in 21 languages*** *– to help smokers quit and to provide information about the health effects of smoking and exposure to tobacco smoke. These resources are free in Victoria and can be purchased by others elsewhere in Australia. Resources are available through the Quit website.* www.quit.org.au/resource-centre/community/ multicultural-project/multicultural-resources.aspx

◆ ***Free information sessions*** *– on the health effects of smoking and second-hand smoking, and information on how to quit. Bilingual educators are available, in a number* of community languages, to attend community groups and English classes.

- **Scholarships** – to health, education and welfare workers fluent in English and in another language to train as Quit educators. Some training participants go on to work with the Multicultural Project and some continue to work with their organisations promoting Quit messages.

- **Community support grants** – these are available each year to support groups or organisations from culturally diverse communities to organise a project that promotes smoke-free messages within their communities.

- **Quitline using the interpreter service** – for people who speak a language other than English and want to talk to a Quit adviser. Callers can contact Quitline 13 7848 and ask for this service or agencies can refer clients using the Multicultural Fax referral available through the Quit website.

- **Working with ethnic media** – including radio, newspapers, ethnic publications and community television to promote information on stopping smoking in a variety of community languages.

- **Brief intervention training for community workers** – Quit Victoria offers brief intervention training for staff in organisations working with CALD communities. Through half-day seminars, the training shows community workers how to help and support smokers from CALD backgrounds to quit.

Visit the Quit website or call Quit on (03) 9635 5502 for more information.

Smoking cessation interventions in the United States that are aimed at ethnic minority people are more acceptable to the ethnic communities involved, but research shows this does not translate into better outcomes. Giving up is hard for everyone. Just keep trying.

Previous education

◆ The potential role of previous education is really interesting. If you examine brains after people have died, you can see 'neurodegeneration' (death of cell structures) and vascular damage (damaged blood vessels that caused damage to tissues), whether or not the person had dementia symptoms while alive. The amount of damage may be the same, no matter how much previous education the person had. The fascinating finding is that if the person did have a lot of formal education they could suffer quite a lot of cell death and vascular damage while still not having dementia symptoms. So studying and becoming highly educated does not stop you getting Alzheimer's disease or vascular disease, but they will help you to cope with that damage happening inside your skull if it does. Margaret Thatcher, the former British Prime Minister, with her two degrees and her busy mental life did get dementia, but arguably she would have been much worse much sooner if she'd left school at age eleven. Recent research indicates that her poor sleep pattern, as little as four hours a night, may have caused her harm. Her highly developed and well-used brain was able to compensate for the damage for longer than others might. The same may be true of other famous people who developed dementia, such as Ronald Reagan.

More education did not protect individuals from developing neurodegenerative and vascular neuropathology by the time they died but it did appear to mitigate the impact of pathology on the clinical expression of dementia before death. The findings suggest that an understanding of the mechanisms leading to functional protection in the presence of pathology may be of considerable value to society. (Professor Carol Brayne)[*]

Exercise

◆ It is well known that exercise reduces stress, boosts your mood and increases energy, but you may not realise that it actually appears to increase the physical amount of grey matter in your brain. The evidence for this in the research literature is very strong, much stronger than the evidence for some of the other suggested interventions here. If you take exercise, even in middle age, it reduces the dementia risk and improves your scores if you have MCI. It protects your brain and slows the decline and reduces the risk of those mini-strokes that cause vascular dementia.

◆ When thinking of a sport to take part in, avoid boxing or anything that involves repeatedly banging your head, like heading a heavy soccer ball. The researchers argue about whether it is the contact with

[*] See C. Brayne et al., 'Education, the Brain and Dementia: Neuroprotection or Compensation?', *Brain*, 133 (2010), pp. 2210–16.

the ball, or repeated clashes where players bang their heads together that causes the problem. Either way, mind your head. Older adults who have had even relatively mild brain injury have an increased risk of dementia. There is no evidence that a single mild injury increases the risk, but the more severe it is and the more repeated, the greater the risk. It might even be that some people have a genetic predisposition to this connection between a bang on the head and dementia. Wear your helmet when cycling. The effects of boxing have been known long enough to have a medical name 'dementia pugilistica'. Surely a head blow in boxing should incur a foul penalty, if we can't ban boxing altogether. Rugby and American football at times seem foolishly dangerous, especially for developing brains, and particularly if young athletes are tempted by the prospect of money, promotion or misplaced team loyalty to keep playing after a concussion. Military personnel also appear to be at risk.

◆ Balance and coordination exercises are useful for all older people if you want to avoid the experience of falling and perhaps sustaining a fracture that will get you admitted to hospital. People with MCI may have greater balance and coordination problems than the general population. Yoga and tai chi seem to work well for improving these functions. In vascular dementia, problems with walking or balancing can occur at an earlier stage than in Alzheimer's. Starting from a higher level of fitness will help you to cope with any deterioration.

◆ Exercise does not need to be solitary or violent. Half an hour five days a week could make a difference. It need only be of moderate intensity. The exercise you are most likely to keep up is the exercise that you enjoy. Socializing is really important also, so if you can combine the two that's great. Think of dancing. You socialise, you take exercise and with a bit of luck, you get a glass of wine. Gardening is also good for you as it provides both exercise and the chance to be outside in daylight or even sunshine, depending on where you live.

◆ Oxygen is the fuel for your brain and if your blood supply is at all compromised, then it is well worth doing anything you can to improve the circulation of your blood and its quality. If you make your heart and blood system more efficient, it will make your brain more efficient. Exercise can do that. Also consider the air quality in your home. Stuffy is bad.

◆ Exercise is magic for avoiding most health problems. Not managing those problems, like blood pressure, makes it more likely that you'll get dementia. There is even a suggested link between obesity and dementia, so get moving in any way that you can, as the exercise will help with weight loss. As many as half of the cases of vascular dementia occur in people with high blood pressure, and exercise reduces your blood pressure. Small studies have indicated that taking blood pressure tablets reduces the risk of dementia, even in Alzheimer's disease.

One woman who corresponded with me was scathing about our support of exercise as a preventive, describing how unwell her husband is with dementia, even though he was a professional athlete. It was important to explain that exercise is only one element of prevention. But later she revealed that he had been a soccer player, and the combination of 'heading' a heavy wet leather ball and a history of subsequent alcohol use told a different story. (Dementia nurse)

Diet

◆ In studies, people who ate the Mediterranean way were less likely to develop dementia. A 'Mediterranean' diet is one that is rich in nuts, fish and vegetables. It should contain plenty of fresh produce and less high-fat dairy and red meat than we have been accustomed to take. It is not clear what the connection is between this diet and dementia, unless it is related to improvements in blood pressure and vascular health. There is no one lifestyle change or dietary change that will eliminate the risk. We need to eat a combination of good food in addition to the other interventions to stay well.

◆ Fibre is famous for reducing constipation and constipation can make you confused, particularly if you are already vulnerable to confusion because you've got some Alzheimer's or vascular damage. Fibre is found only in food that comes from plants. There are two types: soluble and insoluble. Soluble fibre can be digested by your body and helps to reduce the amount of cholesterol in your bloodstream. Your body makes cholesterol out of the fat that you eat. Cholesterol is the building material for the fatty gunk that closes down your blood vessels and irritates the lining of your vascular system, making clots more likely. Clots and narrow blood vessels eventually give rise to blockages and death of brain tissue, and even before that the oxygen supply is being limited. You don't want that. Insoluble fibre is meant to make you feel less hungry for longer, but even when that does not work, at least it keeps your bowels healthy if you take lots of water with it, and it will help you lose weight as part of a healthy lifestyle. (To be honest, even a buttered bread roll filled with French fries could help as part of a healthy lifestyle. The secret is portion control.)

My dad hurt his back and had to take some painkillers. They made him constipated and his bowels got blocked. We did not realise what was happening but he ended up in great pain and it turned out he had not passed water for ten hours. He was retaining urine and had to have a catheter in to empty his bladder. Because he did not drink enough and the catheter was not kept clean he got a urine infection. By the time I got to the apartment you could smell the pee from the door and he was roaring in pain and confusion. He went from mildly demented to completely mad in three days. (Daughter of Roger, 82)

◆ We do need some fat, but because our bodies make cholesterol out of the fat we eat, too much can lead to high cholesterol. Research shows that eating artificial stuff called 'trans fat' (trans-unsaturated fatty acids) is linked to coronary heart disease. You find trans fats in oil that has been industrially hardened and used for frying or for processed foods. It appears in commercial biscuits, cakes and pastries. There is naturally occurring trans fat, but it is in small quantities in any foods like meat or dairy so it is not so harmful. Use liquid oil for frying at home and avoid commercially fried foods if you want to keep your blood vessels unblocked. Early in 2015 the US Food and Drug Administration banned the use of trans fat in food, giving manufacturers three years to comply because they say it is not 'generally recognised as safe'.

◆ Saturated fats are found in fatty meat, butter and lard, sausages and pies, cheeses and cream, and some commercial savoury snacks (such as beef jerky) and chocolate. Recent research by McMaster University in Ontario, Canada was unable to find a clear association between saturated fats and vascular disease. In the developed world we still probably eat too much of these; apart from the question of whether it is narrowing the blood vessels, it can make us overweight, which is hazardous in itself.

◆ Using unsaturated fat instead of saturated or trans fats can help lower blood cholesterol. You find it in oily fish, nuts and seeds, avocados and in sunflower and olive oils. You can also reduce the amount of fat by the cooking methods that you use, eating less 'fast food' and checking the labels on cans and packaging. No single food or nutrient causes or prevents much, but being thoughtful about what you eat is really important.

◆ Oily fish is rich in omega-3 fatty acids. I once suggested that this is good for the brain in a newspaper interview and got an angry letter from a scientist saying that there was not strong enough evidence of dementia-related benefits from omega-3 for him to be persuaded to change his diet on my recommendation. In truth, some studies say yes and some say no. Everyone's grandmother used to call fish 'brain food'. But it has been suggested that if you eat too much fish containing contaminants such as dioxins and polychlorinated biphenyls (PCBs)* you will make yourself ill, so it's recommended for adults that you limit yourself to four portions a week. Omega-3 has been described as anti-atherogenic, anti-inflammatory, antioxidant, anti-amyloid, neuroprotective (these words mean basically that it stops your blood vessels laying down fat and it stops the sort of brain damage that comes from fatty deposits and inflammation of the brain). Is this a wonder food? The research shows that omega-3 is associated with better brain health without actually proving that it causes better brain health. Researchers say that more research is needed. They would, wouldn't they!

---

* The Food Standards Agency has pointed out that these chemicals pollute our waters and are concentrated in the fat stores of fish, so it recommends that adults should eat at least two but no more than four portions of fish a week, and vary the species. Potentially childbearing women and girls have lower limits.

◆ The danger of salt for your heart is well known, but studies have shown that older people who take too much salt and not enough exercise have reduced cognitive power. A teaspoonful a day is too much. When taste buds are dulled by age there is a temptation to pile on the salt to get some more flavour, but that's a bad idea.

◆ Green tea apparently has the same chemicals that are in red wine, chemicals that block the formation of clumps in the brain in Alzheimer's. There is also a suggestion from the research that a cup of coffee can make a positive difference in some people.

◆ You can find more about eating and drinking in Chapter 10.

Vitamins

My uncle is a retired doctor and every morning he takes a folic acid tablet, walks to the shop for his newspaper and then does the crossword, and says, 'Right, that's me without dementia for another day!' (Charlotte, talking about John, 79)

◆ Studies have shown that lower vitamin D concentrations in the blood are associated with poorer cognitive function and a higher risk of Alzheimer's disease. You can get it from food, but even countries like my native Scotland where it is seldom sunny for long we get most of our vitamin D from exposure to sunlight, which allows us to manufacture it ourselves. You'd have to eat a lot of oily fish or take a supplement to get the equivalent of ten minutes in the sunshine. It is also in eggs, and some margarine-type spreads are fortified with it, as are some breakfast cereals. But sunlight is best, particularly in the summer months, when the rays are the right wavelength. Lots of people with dementia, particularly in care homes, never get outside at all. That's not clever.

◆ There has been research in which people with MCI took very large quantities of vitamin B and it seemed to slow down their decline, and fewer of them went on to develop dementia. You'd need to take those vitamins in such large quantities that you'd be best to ask your doctor before embarking on this too enthusiastically. People with a low blood level of folic acid (which is part of the B complex of vitamins) can have dementia-like symptoms and that is why your doctor should test you for this if you complain about your memory.

Mental stimulation

◆ If you don't use it, you lose it! Learning something new is good for your brain. It is like a 'keep fit' regime would be for your heart. The more you use your brain, the better it is for you. You develop a sort of spare capacity that will stand you in good stead if some of your brain tissue starts to shrink or fails because the blood supply has been compromised. Brain scans of people who have learned a lot about something show an increase in the amount of brain tissue they have. For example, in London, England cab drivers have to memorise street names and routes in order to pass an exam before they get a licence. It is called 'the Knowledge' and you see student taxi drivers cruising round London, often on motor scooters, studying street maps. These taxi drivers show a real physical increase in the amount of brain tissue in the hippocampus, a specific region of the brain.

Only a few studies have shown direct evidence for plasticity in the adult human brain related to vital functions such as memory, so this new work makes an important contribution. (Dr John Williams, head of neuroscience at the Wellcome Trust)

◆ In general, if you have more brain capacity, it appears that you can resist the effects of loss of brain cells for longer, but I don't know if cab drivers in London get less dementia than other people. More research is needed, though we already know that the hippocampus is one of the first areas of the brain to be affected by Alzheimer's disease. We also know that both physical exercise and brain exercise can slow shrinkage and even reverse it. Those drivers need to get out and walk when they are off duty.

◆ Enjoy games and puzzles that make you think. Sudoku is very popular for those of us who can't do crossword puzzles. Magazine racks always have stacks of word-search puzzle books and you can buy brain-training programmes to run on your computer, tablet or smart phone. These are so much fun they can end up being mildly addictive. The research on this is variable (just like most of the research). Some people think that if you practice this sort of thing, the main effect is that you get better at the specific puzzle, rather than improving your total brain power, but others are firmly convinced of the benefits. I'm in the latter camp.

◆ Vary your habits. Don't live life on automatic pilot, doing the same thing all the time. Challenge yourself with something new every day of your life. Explore, read, talk to people and find things out. If you develop dementia a whole lot of life will start to become challenging, so practice facing challenges now. Learn how to customise your cellphone, or to use Skype, or set the date and time on the answering machine. Go to town by a different route. Take evening classes.

Quality sleep

◆ Good sleep seems to predispose to the delay of dementia symptoms, and dementia itself is unspeakably tiring, for both the person with dementia and caregivers. So a good sleep schedule is vital.

◆ Chapter 9 (pages 231–2) has ideas on how you can make the bedroom the best it can be for inducing sleep by making simple design changes and using easily available technology, while Chapter 7 (pages 179–80) has some strategies for managing nocturnal wandering.

◆ Sleep is influenced by a hormone in your body called melatonin. Melatonin is produced by a gland in the brain in response to darkness. Its production is inhibited by light and it has a role in setting the body clock. Blood levels are lower in older people and even lower in people with dementia. You can stimulate the metabolism of melatonin by exposing your eyes to daylight, especially in the morning. If you want to sleep tonight, get lots of bright light falling on your retina in the early part of the day. The melatonin slows down bodily functions at night and makes you sleepy. These are two sleep-related reasons for going for a walk in daylight: one is to make you physically tired and the other is to set your body clock with melatonin so that you go to sleep at the same time as most other people where you live. The vitamin D production is a bonus, because it helps reduce falls, apart from any cognitive benefits it brings. In some countries medicinal melatonin is available from pharmacies or doctors. This includes Canada, the United States and Hong Kong.

◆ Smart naps: there is a phenomenon called 'sun-downing' when the person with dementia starts to get irritable and restless in the late afternoon. It has been speculated that this is related to changes in the light level, but more people now think that it is really mainly caused by fatigue, so an afternoon nap might be a good idea.

◆ Sleep is also easier when you are tired.

Mom always did a lot of housework, and now when we don't know what to do, we find some housework for her to do. She polishes brass, irons shirts, cleans floors. Of course she is slow and not very accurate, but it keeps her calm and busy. She sleeps better at night when she's been busy.

(Daughter of Janice, 62)

Stress management and daily relaxation

No one can get inner peace by pouncing on it. (Harry E. Fosdick, American pastor)

◆ Stress can make you look as if you have dementia when you don't. If you have MCI stress can make your symptoms worse. If you have the underlying disease in your brain that causes dementia you might not have any symptoms at all, until stress brings them out. Stress is very, very bad for people with dementia. The stress can make the symptoms so bad that the person may not be able to cope at home. Reducing stress reduces the need for medication.

◆ Practice breathing. Breathing seems so very simple. You inhale and exhale, taking in oxygen and getting rid of carbon dioxide. Your body is really clever and regulates the speed of breathing according to how much oxygen your muscles and other organs need. After running up the stairs you automatically speed up. Hyperventilation is when you breathe faster than your body needs, and it is almost exclusively caused by tension and worry. Other breathing problems occur when you take lots of little inhalations that don't fill your lungs. The fresh air doesn't get as far as the deep pockets of your lungs, where the exchange of oxygen happens. You take lots of shallow breaths without getting much of the precious stuff into your bloodstream. Most of your bodily functions work automatically and you can't control them. It's hard to slow your heartbeat by thinking about it, and you can't consciously regulate how fast urine is made. But you can take charge of your breathing. Slower breathing can lead to relaxation. We all know that, but there's science and body chemistry behind it. Walking slowly can lead to deeper and slower breathing, so a slow walk can help relaxation, and relaxation exercises often focus on tensing and relaxing muscles in turn while controlling breathing. There's evidence of how this helps with a wide range of health care issues, from diabetes to muscle strains.

◆ You can learn a range of relaxation techniques and find one that suits you. You may have tried yoga or tai chi, but there are some that don't need classroom instruction. 'Mindfulness' is the ability to remain aware of how you are feeling right now. You don't think about the past or worry about the future. By staying calm and in the moment, you can reduce the feelings of stress that might overwhelm you. For mindfulness meditation you need to choose a secluded place, indoors or out, where you won't be interrupted. Sit comfortably and focus on an object in your surroundings or close your eyes. Don't worry if distracting thoughts go through your mind, but just turn yourself back to your point of focus. 'Visualisation' is a practice where you close your eyes and imagine a restful scene and then explore it in huge detail, imagining all the sensory experiences you are having in that scene, including sound and touch. You can learn how to use these techniques on your own and they are practical for a busy person to undertake in their own home. Look for tapes and books that you can buy or find information online. The English NHS offers Stress Busters advice on the NHS Choices website (www.nhs.uk). The American Institute of Stress has some good videos that may help; see www.stress.org.

◆ Religious observance is of crucial importance to some people but may become harder to continue in the circumstances that come with dementia and caring. Having a religious belief is associated with lower stress levels, and it is clear that engaging in familiar and safe practices like singing and attending worship can give great comfort. There is still further research to be done on whether religious belief has a positive effect on health, but it is clear that for many people, including caregivers, an opportunity to practice their faith is important for reducing stress. How dementia is 'framed' or perceived in the mind of any human is shaped by their attitude to life, personality, their belief in a soul, or personhood ... and knowing how someone perceives this is very important for understanding how to reduce their stress. Dementia might be perceived as a punishment from a deity for some previous sin or wickedness, or accepted as something to be borne on a journey to paradise. How people think of death and dying is crucial in this space and benefit or damage can occur depending on how we respond to the spiritual or religious needs of the person. You may have to be the Jewish lady singing Christian hymns to comfort a lady with dementia (https://www.youtube.com/watch?v=_chOk04TFaM) or you may be an atheist, reassuring someone that their god will not forget them.

Malcolm Goldsmith, a priest with an interest in dementia, wrote *In a Strange Land* still the finest book on dementia and religious faith. He examines questions from a Christian perspective. People ask, 'Why me? Is this God's punishment?' They wrestle with ethical issues about the belief systems of those giving care. 'As a doctor, can I pray with my patient?' Malcolm offers practical and supportive answers. Here I first read about the American nun Sister Laura. She feared that she was going to forget Jesus because of dementia, and she said to the founding investigator of the Nun Study, David Snowdon, 'I finally realised that I may not remember Him, but He will remember me.'

All religions respect older people. The Quran recognises the effect of dementia in older people. It speaks of how some are 'sent back to a feeble age, so that they know nothing after having known much' and tells us that we must be kind to parents, and 'say not to them a word of contempt, nor repel them, but address them in terms of honour ... even as they cherished me in childhood.' Caring for your ageing parents is incumbent on Muslims. The role of religion in dementia care, and in making people contented is very important.

Active social life

◆ Volunteer! There are so many reasons for volunteering that it deserves a book of its own. Making a difference to other people, having fun, keeping up your skills, making friends … and you can learn new things. People once thought of volunteers as 'do-gooders' who help other people by giving of themselves for no reward. In fact you can't escape the reward, even if you won't take any money for what you do. You are not filling a gap left by someone else who ought to be doing this; you are giving something extra that makes a difference, something that would not be possible without you. Be sure to work for an organisation that offers proper induction and supervision, and ask about expenses. You've got skills that you can pass on. How many young people can you teach to bake, or to run a decent allotment, or to keep chickens?

There is such a fashion for keeping chickens now. They do evening classes and sell books on the subject. We always had chickens when I was a girl, and it has been great fun buying some and showing the grandchildren how to make a bit of money selling eggs. They are amazed at what I know. (Anne, age 82)

◆ Join a club. If you pick the right club you can indulge in your interest. If you are boring your family and friends to death with your knowledge of steam locomotives, imagine the pleasure of being with others who will talk about it until long after everyone else has ceased to be interested. Bliss. Socializing is good for delaying dementia symptoms and reducing them. No one is sure why, but who cares if it means you get to see newly discovered pictures of the Flying Scotsman? A book club will encourage you to read books that you would not normally choose, and even if you are only listening to others discussing the issues that arise from the books it can stimulate your thinking. The issues in a good book are universal and eternal and you can join in a discussion of those issues from your life experience, even if your recent memories are a bit hazy.

◆ Taking classes is a good idea, even though it is often said that people with dementia can't learn new things. You can live in the moment, enjoying the experience, without having to worry about tests and exams. An example is a class run in Melbourne, Australia, by the National Gallery of Victoria that is specifically for people with dementia. The programme has been developed to tap into the imagination of people with dementia through multiple workshops and visits to the gallery. Art triggers both the mind and the emotions and, of course, if you take lots of classes before you get dementia, it can delay the onset. Education, brain training – call it what you like. It is probably the social aspect that makes the biggest difference. Anyone going to the pub later? The Dementia Festival of Ideas in 2015 explored the impact of the arts and culture on dementia and turned a spotlight on ten creative ideas from across the world that will help caregivers and people with dementia, in ways that might delay symptoms in some cases; visit www.dementia.stir.ac.uk/ideas/ideaslab-2015#jessica

◆ Keeping connected with family and friends offers great health benefits. It could be that just keeping tabs on them is a significant mental exercise that keeps the grey matter active.

We've got two children and six grandchildren and one great-granddaughter, and one is retired and three are working, and we've had two weddings in the last five years. And the new baby. And the grandchildren are working in England and New Zealand, so we have to write to them and talk on the phone. The grandson lost his job ... he was really worried for a while, so we kept phoning him ... [Laughs] It's a full-time job just remembering the birthday cards, never mind everything else! I have to keep a book and mark it all on the calendar. (Grandmother, 85)

◆ Some people don't have big families and rely even more on friends. You need to make dates and get out and keep seeing them as much as you can. Research shows that the stimulation you get does not have to be as highbrow as doing the crossword in the *New York Times*. Ladies who go to bingo (a much-maligned simple betting game) are in better cognitive shape than those who stay at home. The complexities of organizing your transport, your pals, the money and just getting there are a challenge in themselves, never mind keeping an eye on the numbers. The best socializing is whatever you enjoy most, because that is what you will keep up, and it is persevering that makes a difference.

Is there a miracle cure?

When you surf the Internet looking for ideas about what makes a difference in dementia, you'll find a lot of information out there. There have been stories about coconut oil and turmeric, ginkgo biloba and vitamin supplements, cow's milk colostrum and pansies, and a whole range of nutritional advice that is supposed to improve brain function. My problem with all of these is that they may send people off on a wild-goose chase. The stressed and anxious buyer under pressure will spend money that they can't afford on things whose benefits are not proven, with side effects they were not warned about. They are not helped by the way in which research is undertaken and how it is reported in sensational terms in the media. From day to day 'miracles' are celebrated and then disproved. It is hard at times to know what to do for the best, because at some point it might be discovered that one of these really works.

However, there is no escaping the fact that at the moment the intervention for which there is the greatest evidence of effectiveness is exercise, along with socializing and keeping active in any way that you can.

chapter 7

Disturbing behaviours

Most of the time, things will be just as they always were. You are living with the same person. However, the dementia will at some stage make the person you know behave in new ways that cause you and them stress and distress. This chapter will help you with ideas for avoiding that sort of disturbing behaviour and suggest ways of dealing with it together. People with dementia say they get irritated when they are treated in a different way by those they live with, above all in the early stages of their condition, so remember that your husband, wife, parent or other loved one is still for a lot of the time the person they were yesterday.

When we came out of the clinic and they'd told me it was dementia I was in shock. It was an even bigger shock when I realised my wife wouldn't even let me take the rubbish out in case I got lost. (Don, 73)

Sadly, later in the journey, people with dementia may eventually present problems from time to time, both to themselves and to their families when they are living together, because of behaviour that other people find upsetting. You will not experience all of these tribulations, and if they do happen they are unlikely to be a permanent feature. As dementia progresses, symptoms come and go. Research has shown that there are six areas that present the greatest test for caregivers. These are:

- aggression;
- agitation or anxiety;
- depression;
- hallucinations and delusions;
- sleeplessness;
- wandering.

Medication has only a limited role in dealing with any of these. If the person is on dementia-specific medication, it helps. The other medications that doctors might prescribe include sedatives that may not work and can have bad side effects. Others, like non-sedative antidepressants, can be useful in anxiety and depression, but the fewer drugs one has to take the better. In this chapter I am going to suggest non-drug responses to each of these six challenges based on the original advice in the booklet *10 Helpful Hints for Carers*. These are strategies that you can try on your own at home that we know from research or experience can make a difference. Of course, you may try all of them and find they don't work. At that stage you really need professional help.

Remember that some people, including dementia professionals, don't like the words that are used to name this behaviour. People with dementia have been denigrated in the past and the words used to describe them have had to be changed to show more respect. For example, in English, the word 'senile' technically only means 'characteristic of old age' but it is a very offensive word now if it is used about a person with dementia because it is used to mean 'decaying' or 'decrepit'. Expressions like 'disturbing' and 'wandering' are starting to be regarded as offensive in the same way, for similar reasons. We know that disturbing behaviour is caused by stress and distress, and some professionals prefer to call it 'distressed' behaviour because that high-lights the fact that the real problem is not that we are disturbed, but that the other person is distressed. While these changes in language take hold, we all need to be able to understand both expressions, and use them sensitively, because understanding what we are each talking about is a very high priority. We don't need to fall out about it.

Aggression

An important note is that if your relationship is with someone who was always violent, this is a different and difficult case and you need to ask for help at once. Start with your doctor. Frontotemporal dementia, the one that affects the front of the brain, can give rise to aggression, because the frontal lobes of the brain are the place where your inhibitions lie. That brain damage makes it harder to control impulses. The psychiatric team or the doctor can tell you about this in advance so that you can anticipate problems and let the team know if and when they become an issue. In other sorts of dementia it can occur simply because of what is going on. Aggression does not occur in every person with dementia, and generally that is only for a short time, but it is always shocking, because it is most likely to hurt those who are trying to help. You can approach this problem in a number of ways.

◆ Leave the room. It is imperative to keep yourself out of harm's way. Giving the person time and space to calm down is helpful. You remove any possible annoyance that you personally have innocently caused and it means that you are safer. The proverb says 'Sticks and stones will break my bones, but names will never hurt me'. However, this is not strictly true. Even verbal aggression will affect your well-being, so give yourself a break. Walking away also removes you from the understandable but completely unacceptable temptation to hit back. It gives both parties time and space to calm down, and allows you time to work out who you can turn to. It is not your fault but the result of the condition, and do not be afraid to ask for help, even if you think what is happening is shameful.

I woke up and found my husband beside the bed brandishing a knife. He said, 'What have you done with my wife, you evil bitch. I don't know who you are, but you better get out of here!' (Edith, 79)

It is worth saying at this point that if you live in a country where guns are readily available, now is the time to get rid of any weapons around the home. Don't tempt fate.

◆ It is really very tough, but do everything in your power not to argue with a person who has dementia. There is no point and it will create an atmosphere that will make things worse. Even if you manage to convince them that the thought they have is wrong, they may forget that position very soon and start back on the old tack. The problem is that people with dementia get a sort of emotional hangover, where they feel angry and suspicious long after the occurrence that caused those feelings. Try to avoid 'No, but …' and replace it with 'Yes, and …' If you don't you may inadvertently create more trouble for yourself.

Mr Smith was a gentle and devoted husband with one hobby, betting on the horses on a Saturday. His wife had always kept the family finances, so he asked her for money for his bet once a week. When dementia set in he started asking for the money randomly, and more than once a day. If she argued that he'd had it, or it was not Saturday, he got really angry and rough with her. She could not give him money every time he asked because he frequently hid it, lost it or gave it away, and it could be up to fifty or sixty dollars a day. The son came up with a great solution: persuading his mother not to argue but to hand out a reproduction old-style ten-dollar note (badly copied to avoid fear of forgery accusations, the sort that is used as a stage prop) every time Mr Smith asked. The only people who complained were the grandchildren, who sometimes got given them for their allowance. He never actually did go out to the bookies. He just needed to know he could whenever he wanted, because to him it is always Saturday. She just stopped arguing. (Dementia nurse)

◆ Check if the person is in pain. Undiagnosed and untreated pain is one of the common causes of disturbing behaviour in dementia. Even if they are not complaining of pain it might be at the root of the behaviour. Your doctor can help with this. If swallowing pills is an issue, consider transdermal patches – pain patches that are put on like a Band-Aid or adhesive dressing and deliver slow-release analgesia through the skin.

◆ Work out if there are any noticeable triggers for the disturbing behaviour. Aggression may be a coherent response from a person who misinterprets what is happening because of deficits in their understanding and recall. They know something is wrong and they are angry and scared, so they fight. If you see the world from their point of view, you'll understand why it actually makes sense to fight. If they've always been confident and competent and everything seems to be going wrong, they might do something extreme. As the person tries to work out where they are and what is going on, they make mistakes. Is this a bathroom or a storeroom? Is the person trying to undress them a nurse or a rapist? The violent resistance to being cared for is logical within the world view of a person who cannot remember or work things out and may be experiencing hallucinations. There are design ideas in Chapter 9 that might help with this. Keep a diary about the person's moods and get a sense of what sets them off and what they find relaxing and comforting. You are going to have to talk to professionals about this and details of what happens and when will help them work out how they can help you and assess the level of risk that you have.

My mother suddenly decided she disliked baths and my dad was able to muddle through until she had a bad fall. When she came back from hospital for a while nurses came in to help with washing – it was a disaster. Mum got aggressive and called the Nigerian nurse a 'darkie', much to my dad's shame. I can understand that you don't want strangers manhandling you, but basic hygiene is important. We're still wrestling with this one. (Ruth, whose mother has dementia)

◆ Consider taking the person for a walk and offer as much opportunity for activity as possible. Fresh air and exercise can help with mood and natural fatigue reduces stress. You might be starting to wonder if I believe that exercise solves everything, but to be honest it has amazing value. The person with dementia will find it harder to fight if they are tired. Although some people get irritable when tired, it's possible that a long walk will make them more likely to nap than snap.

◆ Try to avoid future outbursts by creating a calm environment. There is advice on this later in this chapter. How you do it will be different for every individual. Find out what works and keep doing it.

◆ Make life less challenging. If you start to forget how to use everyday objects the frustration is maddening. People with dementia sometimes become disinhibited, and where once they would have gritted their teeth, they may now just lose their self-control. Fear leads to violence.

◆ Touch and comforting words that work when the person is anxious may also work to ward off aggression, but make sure that the touch is not misunderstood as restraint, because the person will attempt to get away, perhaps hurting you and themselves in the process.

Agitation or anxiety

A range of issues can generate agitation in a person with dementia, so you have to be a detective and find out what usually causes it in this person in order to avoid those triggers. Anything bothering a person with dementia gets intensified because they've lost the capacity to distract themselves or to move away from what is upsetting them. Their behaviour may be restless or clingy, and they may cry out.

◆ Protect yourself from the strain that arises when you are living with an agitated person. If they are inconsolable for long periods it will give rise to strong feelings in you, such as anger, frustration or resentfulness. You might start to feel hopeless about the situation. You need to take breaks away and to keep up your own emotional, social and spiritual supports as much as you can.

She kept crying out for her mother who died before we were married. It was really difficult for me. In a way, I felt like joining her and crying out for my mother. In the end I could hardly stand it. (Husband of Jane, 64)

◆ See if there is an underlying physical problem. Does the agitated person have pain or an unmet need, such as hunger or thirst? You might take them to the doctor to see if there is any undiagnosed clinical condition.

◆ As we have seen, touching and holding can really help, as long as the person does not think you are trying to restrain them. In agitation the person has an overwhelming feeling that they need to get away and their body is flooded with 'flight or fight' hormones, so if you restrain them you are restricting their choice and all that's left is 'fight'. If you have never tried massage, now is the time. The combination of a peaceful setting, restful music, perhaps candlelight and scented oils, and the comfort from the physical touch to loosen knotted muscles can really help. If you are not up to that, just rubbing someone's hands or feet with moisturiser or stroking their hair may help, if they will let you.

◆ The agitated person might pace about and so you can use up some of this energy with purposeful exercise:

Dad used to get in a right state cooped up in the house. I'd get him out in the garden and ask him to help me dig the potato patch. We never put any potatoes in there, but it got a good digging over and he seemed more relaxed after. (Son, speaking about his retired father, who had been a garbage collector)

◆ Aromatherapy has been the subject of serious
research in dementia. No one quite knows why it
works. The person with dementia, particularly if
they are very old, has a reduced sense of smell, so
researchers think it's not necessarily the nice smell
that makes it work. Lemon balm and lavender have
produced significant reductions in agitated behaviour,
including sleeplessness and wandering. It seems not
only to be the personal attention or massage that
makes the difference, because essential oils work
better than vegetable oil. It has been wondered if the
reduced agitation is a result of the calming effect on
the carer of administering this pleasant treatment.
Worth a try, but make sure that you follow the
instructions for use of essential oils.

◆ A calming atmosphere can help a lot. It is most
soothing for a person at home if as little as possible is
changed. You may make some small changes so that
the place is safer under foot, removing trip hazards,
in order to avoid falls that could lead to a hospital
admission.

◆ Because the person does not remember the passage
of time, they may start to look for lost possessions.
You might agree one day to replace an old chair and
then the person starts to look for it again the following
day and wonder what's happened to it. We all forget
things like this from time to time, but in dementia
because it happens so often the person might be
made agitated by the constant sense that something is
changing without their control. How many of us say

from time to time, 'I could have sworn I had another …' when we've forgotten that we used up the last one? That is normal. In dementia you may have to handle more fundamental forgetting.

I'm sure the toilet used to be here. (Jack, 85, pointing to the cupboard under the stairs)

It's important not to add to the anxiety by arguing, but distraction can make a difference. Jack's daughter can say, 'Well, here it is now, behind this other door.' And putting a clear label on the toilet door or leaving the door open for the toilet to be seen is a good way of distracting the person from looking for it fruitlessly in the wrong place.

◆ People who have agitation sometimes seem to benefit from light therapy or daylight lamps. These are meant to have the same effect as being outside in daylight, because they give off the same spectrum of light. Walking in the open air would be even better, but sometimes this is not practical. Keep the house as full of light as possible, using the design ideas listed in Chapter 9. Daylight lamps are also said to help with depression.

◆ Music is such good medicine it should be available through insurance. However, just as you need to take the right medicine, so it needs to be the right music. In order to make the correct choice you need to know a lot about the person. Research shows that music still has meaning and a positive effect for a person with dementia and their caregiver up to the very end of life.

Being able to respond to music is the one thing dementia cannot destroy. Playlist for Life encourages families and caregivers to create a playlist of personally meaningful music on an iPod for people with dementia …We've begun developing a Playlist for Life app with Glasgow Caledonian University to deliver a personal music intervention from diagnosis to end of life. It will be informed by robust research evidencing the impact of personal music on the wellbeing of those living with dementia … (http://www. playlistforlife.org.uk/)

◆ There is a movement in dementia care which is called 'life story work'. This means working with the person to find out interesting and important things about their life. What you consider most fascinating may not be what they regard as important to them. For example, you might think that it was most significant that someone was a great army general, but his most memorable experience might be that he wrote and published a children's book. Of course everything from someone's past defines them to an extent, but it's important to go beyond the obvious things that everyone knows about a person and get close to what matters to them. There may be topics they wish to avoid, because they find them painful. On the other hand, people do sometimes find comfort in thinking about the past even if it was sad, and shedding a tear, before going on to think of something else. In general, though, life story work is meant to be fun. Creating a scrapbook is a practical way of working on this, and you end up with something that other people can use to stimulate conversation, or to sit and quietly look through as a distraction when the person is agitated. If you are able to create a digital version of the scrapbook and print it out or share it on a laptop or other device, this will guard against the risk of the material getting lost or destroyed. You can also share that version with relatives all over the world to find out if they have any more reminiscences or ideas or photos to add to the story.

When we were doing dad's memory book, we discovered some photographs of Uncle Alex wearing coveralls and a hat, from the days when he worked on the railroad. Some of the pictures had been cut in half. We asked dad, and he knew it was Alex, but one day he suddenly said, 'That was George … he would have been cut out of the picture. Your grandmother did that.' We asked around a bit and the most the old aunts would tell us was 'Your uncle Alex had a friend on the railway.' Dad died and he never told us what was behind that story. (D, son of Ronald, 92)

For a variety of reasons, some stories will never, ever be shared, but there are treasured memories you can capture now before they are lost.

Depression

◆ Activities that relieve boredom or provide distraction can help with depression. Anyone who is bored or inactive may feel down and fed up. You know this person well, so you know what would cheer them up:

When Mom gets down I stick her in the car and take her down to the shopping mall and we sit in the food court watching the world go by. Then we go round the shoe shops and shock ourselves with the price of shoes and the terrible high heels that girls wear these days. (Son, 60)

◆ A dog or cat is a great companion for people who need cheering up. It does not matter how depressed his owner is, the dog still needs a walk. Fresh air, exercise and daylight will help to combat those low feelings and also be good for the dog. Cats provide companionship in a less demanding way and are easier to keep in many ways, taking themselves out and in through a cat-flap when they need to. And they do remind their owners when they need to be fed. People sometimes ask me if a person with dementia might forget to feed their dog. I suspect the greater danger is that the dog will learn to ask for food more often, on the basis that his owner might forget he's already had some. Dogs are smart.

◆ Remembering the past is a great distraction from depression. When people are losing some of their capacity, you need to be aware that much of the stuff they know from the past will be lost if you don't ask them about it now. Our oral tradition of telling stories is not just about the preservation of the stories but also about the great pleasure of telling them and listening to them, even when they are familiar.

Tell me again, Granny, about when you jumped on top of the wedding cake because they would not let you be a bridesmaid. (A.B., 11)

You need to learn the trick of starting a really good conversation about the past, and take the person out of their gloomy spiral of thoughts.

◆ There is research that suggests you can make things better using 'multisensory therapy', which involves stimulating the person with music and light and even nice smells, to lift them from their depression. You can buy a machine with fibre-optic strands to play with and lights that change their colour. In some care homes they have whole rooms with this equipment. It is often not used, so if there is one, try it out when you are visiting. Because it is hardly ever used, I'd hesitate to install one, but if it is there, have a look.

◆ Although it's wrong to argue, there is a great temptation when someone is depressed to try to correct them about what is getting them down:

The old lady was crying because she'd been told her mother was dead. She cried as if her mother had died yesterday. Her mum died fifty years ago. I heard her husband going on and on at her to remind her that they all went to the funeral before their children were even born. (Dementia nurse)

There is an alternative way of dealing with this raw emotion called 'validation'. Instead of making her out to be wrong, because it would be frightening and depressing to have to comprehend that she is losing her grip on reality on top of the utter sense of bereavement, the best response is to go with the flow of the feelings – which are 'valid' under the circumstances:

I advised him not to tell her again that her mother was long dead. He thought she should know and she'd get over it if she was reminded that it was long ago. Instead I took her to sit on the sofa and put my arm round her and said, 'Oh, your mother was a lovely lady, wasn't she? Was she a good cook? Tell me all about what she is like …' I drifted into the present tense. 'Does she use bones for soup or a stock cube?' (Dementia nurse)

It does not really matter whether she is wrong about when her mother died. The important thing is to offer comfort, because it is right to feel grief or pain when you are missing someone. Most of us feel less pain over time after someone has died. We still love them and their memory, but it does not hurt so much. If you have forgotten that the time has passed, your grief feels very new and it is genuine and should be treated as such. You can't be argued out of it. The solution is gentle distraction. It must be a nightmare to live through these storms of emotion.

When I was training to be a nurse forty years ago I was asked to wake up a man who had alcohol-related brain damage. He was a heavy drinker anyway, but his wife died in a car crash and he drank himself into oblivion. When I went to his room he seemed a bit bewildered. 'Where am I?' 'In hospital.' He swore loud and long and cheerfully. 'What happened? What time is it?' I started to try to tell him that he needed to come for breakfast, but he started grabbing his clothes and shoes to dress quickly. 'She'll be waiting for me off the night shift. Oh, my God, I'll be in trouble.' In a quiet firm voice I told him his wife was dead, he was ill, and he needed to come for breakfast. He would not believe me at first, but when he looked in my face and I repeated it he crumpled up and sobbed. I confessed later to the charge nurse that I felt I had not handled it well, and should have treated it more like breaking bad news than correcting his confusion. 'Never mind,' he sighed. 'I'll give you another shot with him tomorrow morning when he wakes, and each day for the rest of the week.' (Retired psychiatric nurse)

Comfort is needed, not logical argument. Apart from anything else, you may have to go through this a number of times. So you need to make it easy on yourself and the bereaved person. Don't argue about anything. Nothing will be gained on either side, neither insight nor satisfaction.

◆ Many dementia organisations recommend counselling as a help for depression. The research that has been done so far does not suggest that it makes a great difference, but when you see how often it is recommended by those who should know, it must be worth trying. The counsellor needs to know that the client has dementia as some of the commonly used techniques might not work for people with dementia. Some operant conditioning relies on the person having a working memory, and that is not always there. It depends on the definition of counselling, and whether that includes validation therapy, or redirection.

◆ Companionship of other people is hugely important. People with dementia, particularly in the early stages, get great support from joining a group of people like themselves. Contact your local Alzheimer's organisation to find out where there is one or ask the community psychiatric nurse if they are going to start one. Dementia support groups are a great place to talk in safety about subjects that are of concern. Not least, they are a place where people may experience moments of great happiness:

I am a professor in the field and I take it all very seriously. The people in the dementia working group, all of whom have dementia, have me rocking with laughter. It is about dementia, about themselves, about how others treat them. Of course they are angry and sad, but they share their laughter generously and tell me it is better than any medicine. (*from* 10 Helpful Hints for Carers)

◆ As with the person who faces aggression or agitation, the person living with someone who has depression needs to care for themselves as well in order not to be dragged down by the circumstances. If the person you are looking after is beyond consolation, you need to contact someone and your doctor will be the first port of call. Sometimes people with dementia (and their carers) can develop a clinical depressive illness that is more than an ordinary response to the stress of the situation. You need support, which might include medication.

Hallucinations and delusions

A hallucination is the experience of seeing or hearing something that is not really there. In fact you can hallucinate with any of your five senses. It's different from an illusion. I might think I see a face in the pattern on the floor rug, but when I concentrate I can see it is only a carpet. That would be an illusion. A hallucination would be when I see a face in the carpet and there is no pattern or shadow that could explain the mistake. That's more common in Lewy body dementia than in other forms. The brain is constantly trying to make sense of the messages it receives and if it is not working properly it 'invents' something to make sense of the poorly processed information it has.

My dad is tortured with the Lewy body. At night, he'll be shouting and swearing and fighting with enemies that aren't there. He can see them and hear them. And mother is trying to sleep downstairs from him because she's afraid he'll hit her. He doesn't mean it. And in the morning he apologises. Always. It's almost worse that he realises what he's been like. It's a living nightmare. (Son of Mr B., who has Parkinson's disease and Lewy body dementia)

A delusion is a fixed false belief that is contrary to culture and implausible. You might think that your dad already has a number of fixed false beliefs: for example, that his football team might win the league, or that we don't notice his bald patch under the comb-over – these are reasonable bits of self-delusion shared by men in many cultures. Don't go there, because his ideas are almost plausible. However, if he believes unshakably that someone is stealing from him or that your mother is having an affair with the bank manager when clearly she is a frail little grandmother who has only ever loved one man, this is a delusion. It's not credible. It is the result of the disease and you have to decide what to do about it to look after them both. The general rules are about distraction, making sure the person is well and avoiding arguments.

It may be that he has forgotten that he disposed of some cash and is now looking for it and assumes that it must have been stolen. He may be having difficulty remembering how long his wife has been out of the house on an errand and putting two and two together to make five about her absence. There may be something in the past that is surfacing for him. There is no point in trying to get to the bottom of any of that. The most important thing is to stop anyone getting upset, if at all possible.

The issue about culture is important in deciding if something is a delusion. A person with dementia might be said to be deluded because they believe an angel is by their side all day that no one else can see. Before deciding to act upon this, remember that not all delusions are frightening and bad, and this might not even be a delusion for all you know. So you might decide to leave that source of comfort as it is.

One really difficult situation is when the person has a fixed, false belief that they need to go 'home' for some reason. The wail of distress when you tell a mother that she can't go home to her child is real, even if the child is long grown up and gone away. That sort of feeling is a kind of delusion and the most effective response is distraction.

The general rules of thumb for hallucinations and delusions are similar.

◆ It is a good idea not to argue with a person who has dementia, ever. You will probably both continue to believe that the other is wrong and neither of you will like it. Arguing about the existence of the object that is being hallucinated, or the voices or smell or sound, is fruitless. Another way of saying this is that you should not try to 'prove' anything. If your mother hallucinates and thinks small animals surround her chair she'll be distressed if you trample all over the carpet to prove they are not there. She'll be as distressed as she would be if they were real. Her distress will continue long after she's forgotten what you did to upset her. You won't be able to argue your father out of the idea of thieves or infidelity. You can only distract him from his anger and get him out of her way till he forgets it.

So when he started on about her having an affair, I just said, 'Good grief. Have you seen the time? We were supposed to be at the town centre half an hour ago to pick up my nephew.' And I got him into his coat and into the car and we went to a café, and when the nephew did not turn up (which would have been a miracle, because he lives in London now) we had a pot of tea and went home. (Son of Mr B.)

You may have to repeat the distraction exercises. Some delusions stick around for a bit.

◆ If you increase the light level and make everything clear, you can at least reduce the likelihood that the person with dementia is also struggling with illusions.

Another bad day today. I saw my reflection in the lounge plate-glass window after dark and started yelling at Moira that the neighbours were in our garden and that she should call the police. Of course, it turned out to be me. (Gerald, 68)

Because illusions may arise from confusion caused by mirrors and reflections, covering up windows with nets or closing blinds and curtains at night helps. A bright light in the garden at night that might prevent the mirror-like reflections back into the room is another possible strategy.

◆ Fortunately, hallucinations in dementia are not always unpleasant. This is in marked contrast to the hallucinations suffered by people with depression. However, if the image was horrible and frightening, it is better to give comfort than to dismiss the expression of anxiety as unfounded. It has been suggested that the person is more likely to hallucinate if there is not much going on. It appears that some people with dementia hallucinate and are aware of the hallucination but are able to 'tune out' of it. It has been said it's like having the TV on but not watching it; or like having someone talking in the room to whom you are paying no attention. They are still aware of it but they screen it out, which is harder to do if there is nothing much else happening.

◆ Avoid boredom for the same reason. However, it is important to note that stress makes hallucinations more likely. It's tricky. If you over-stimulate or under-stimulate you could add to the problem. Knowing the person really well will help you to judge it right. The symptoms more often strike in the evening. The person may be conscious or drowsy and inaccessible. Hallucinations are usually visual, but a small number of people experience sounds or voices that are not there and some experience smells.

Well, you ask me about distraction? To be honest, it's whatever works. One of my patients can be distracted over and over by the same DVD on the television. Others will refuse to enjoy their usual entertainment when they are disturbed and so a walk outside works best – just to tire them out a bit. Remember that most of us can be distracted by words, or conversation, but the person with dementia may be getting less verbal and more non-verbal. It's whatever works for that individual. The really clever thing is if you can work out what it is that sets them off, and do something about that. (Dementia adviser)

◆ You have to make sure that the person has enough to eat and drink and enough sleep.

◆ You can ask the pharmacist or doctor to review the medication, because some combinations can cause a problem. On the other hand, it might be another physical illness (that can be treated) that is making the situation worse. The doctor may be able to offer medication that might make a difference. There are risks if antipsychotic medication is used, but it can help some people. It might even be that an eye and hearing test would help to prevent the sorts of illusions or misperceptions that precede hallucinations or precipitate delusions:

Mary was sure that the neighbours were prowling round the house at night and she got quite paranoid about it, but the situation improved radically after we'd got her hearing aids and her glasses fixed. (Daughter of Mary, 75)

◆ Some hallucinations can be almost harmless. If they are not getting in the way of daily living, you might not worry about them too much, as long as you've checked with the doctor that there is nothing preventable. Understanding the cause should make you less worried, but make sure you've asked to see if there is anything that can be fixed.

Remember the squirrel:

My mum kept saying to me when I asked her how she was, 'Oh, don't worry about me. Basil keeps me company. He comes round for afternoon tea.' We assumed that she had an imaginary friend because we knew about the hallucinations and delusions and she'd had Parkinson's. I wondered if we should tell the doctor. The children even joined in talking about Basil. When I was doing her blinds one day I saw this squirrel on the washing pole and when I pointed it out to her she said, 'Of course, that's old Basil. Open the window and he'll come in for his treats.' (From 10 Helpful Hints for Carers)

This daughter assumed that there was a hallucination or a delusion when there was neither.

Sleeplessness

When people talk about the stress of caring and the physical illnesses that caregivers suffer, a lot of it may be down to inadequate sleep. It is hard to rest when you have to keep one eye open all night because someone in the house has developed nocturnal behaviours. Sleep deprivation is used as torture, and we all know why.

◆ Here we go again with the exercise advice! If people get exercise they sleep better. It is possible to exercise in the house, with chair exercises and dancing and moving about. But exercise that exposes you to daylight, particularly in the early part of the day, is especially good for you. The reason is explained in Chapter 9 (page 215) in the section on light.

◆ At every stage of life having a bedtime routine is important for getting people to settle. You know what works best in your house. However, it is worth noting the obvious things. Screen time should be stopped an hour or two before settling, because the light stimulation does affect the body clock. Whatever is comforting, like a milky drink or a warm bath, provide these things if you can – make them part of a familiar routine. Everyone should know that when the TV goes off and the cocoa is served it is nearly time to turn in.

◆ Even in some nursing homes now, night-time care workers are being issued with bath robes so that if someone wakes up in the night they are not met with the spectacle of people walking about in daytime clothes. The night attire helps to give an impression that they may disturb other sleepers and they are more receptive to being encouraged back into bed. Putting away daytime objects like clothing and shoes gives visual cues to the fact that it is bedtime.

It's logical to me. I was a nurse all my working life. If I end up in a care home and wake up in the night and see lots of staff milling about in scrubs, I'll probably get up and ask for jobs to do. If our residents get up and see us wearing a robe it is easier to put your finger to your lips and say, 'Shhh! Don't wake everyone up. Let's go back to your room and I'll bring you a nice cup of tea so you can settle down till morning ...' (Jane, 59)

◆ People sleep better in a cool room with a warm bed. Just being too hot can make the person inclined to get up for a wander. If they then see that the outside light is on they may go out to investigate. Better to encourage a quick trip to the toilet before snuggling down again by keeping the room cooler.

When my mother went for respite to the care home the staff made a big issue about her not sleeping but wandering about and they got the doctor to prescribe sleeping pills for it. I was very annoyed and pointed out that the radiator in her room could not be turned down and she was uncomfortable with the unaccustomed heat at night. They said there was nothing that could be done, but I complained to the manager and a heating engineer repaired the control on her radiator that day. It was nonsense. (Hazel, daughter of M., 85)

◆ Talking of light, it is important to keep the room as dark as possible, particularly if this is what the person is used to, or if they are accustomed to a small night-light. Darkness has a physiological effect on the body. In Northern countries, in summer, the daylight creeps in at about 4.30 a.m. – a time to get some blackout blinds. Even moonlight can interfere with sleepiness.

◆ The most common reason for getting out of bed at night is to go to the bathroom. If you have an ensuite bathroom and you can position the bed so that the toilet can be seen when the person's head is on the pillow, that is an ideal arrangement. When using the toilet they can see the comfy bed and when in bed they can see the toilet. The greatest problem is when the person starts to wander round the house looking for, and even forgetting that they are looking for, the bathroom and then being unable to find their way back to bed.

◆ By the time we are old, most of us have developed a variety of aches and pains. Taking a painkiller half an hour before bedtime might mean that those creaky joints and tired muscles don't get in the way of dropping off to sleep. Talk to the doctor about whether over-the-counter medicines are advisable and if they will be enough. We all know the danger of mixing drugs and alcohol, and so it is worth having a discussion with the doctor about this while you are there. A small alcoholic drink might help the person to drop off to sleep. Too much is counterproductive, as anyone who drinks a lot may be wakeful in the early hours when the effects start to wear off. Ask the doctor if a glass of beer or a small sherry would be appropriate at bedtime. (You might need something yourself, and you know that a glass of wine a day helps delay dementia ... so think of it as medicinal!)

My husband wakes up in the middle of the night craving a banana sandwich. Give him that and a slurp of milk and he will drop off to sleep again very quickly. He ought to brush his teeth, but who cares, if it is a choice between that and a better night's sleep for me? I make up the snack in advance to keep it quick and simple. (Wife of C., 62)

◆ When you are at the end of your tether you may consider asking the doctor for a sedative. You have to be careful with them, though, because they can cause a 'hangover' the next day, so the person may be drowsy and more likely to doze, and not take enough exercise or eat enough, which means there may be trouble the next night. If they are dopey it might cause a fall. However, needs must when things get tough.

Wandering

In academic circles there are arguments about what to call 'wandering'. I use this word because it is probably the term that most people use and understand. The reason for wanting to use other words is that the person is not usually drifting around, but heading purposefully for something. Our problem is that we don't know what that purpose is, so it looks like pointless wandering. And even if we find out that the purpose is something futile, such as setting off for work decades after retirement, or popping round to see long-dead friends, or getting down to the school to collect the little ones, who are now grown up and living in Peru, we can still do something that will help.

◆ Step one is to try to work out the purpose. You can gently or casually ask, 'Where are you going? What is it you want? Can I help you?' Start to get a picture of what's usually wanted and you can anticipate it. Maybe there is someone who will take them for a walk every morning right at the time they always want to leave the house? If you are busy and live near a dangerous road you will be tempted to lock the front door or the garden gate. The problem with this is that the person will probably redouble their efforts to get out and they'll become angry and frustrated – feelings that may be taken out on you. This is where being able to anticipate the problem and make a plan will help.

◆ Exercise is a potential solution to many problems. Whatever the reason for wanting to wander, a person is less likely to do it if they are physically tired. If they have an overwhelming sense that they want to go somewhere, then getting the right clothes and shoes on and getting someone to go with them is good. As people with dementia are often older and frailer, a diverting walk with an offer to return home for a cup of tea and a sit-down after is often enough to calm them and in the end takes up less time than arguing about it all day.

◆ The kinds of ideas that would give rise to anxiety and the need to get out are less likely to occur if the person with dementia is busy and occupied. Boredom and frustration go hand in hand. Your house is not a holiday camp and you need to do chores and live your own life, but planning for some distractions can be really helpful:

I got a box set of episodes of Cheers. *To be honest, I could have just bought one disc, because he is happy to watch it over and over. Just hearing the theme tune starting again is enough to get him to get into his chair and settle down.*
(Wife of Rex, 82)

◆ When judging a UK Design Council competition recently I was introduced to the 'dementia dog'. This was originally thought of as a career-change opportunity for dogs who failed the practical at 'dogs for the blind' training. These companion animals are a great idea. The dog needs walking and wears a vest that tells the world that he is looking after his master. Unlike dogs for the blind, which have to be respected and not petted when they are working, this animal is an invitation to stop and talk. They can also be trained to respond to a timer in the house by fetching a bag with medicine in it when the timer goes off to remind you to take your medication. And if you give the order 'Home!' it can help overcome that problem of returning to the wrong house. Canine caregivers offer a wide range of benefits to their owner. A non-profit in the United States called Dog Wish (www.dogwish.org) presents a short film about Rick, who has dementia, and his service dog, Sam, who alerts him to pots being neglected on the stove by barking loud and continuously until Rick switches the stove off. The dog, when resting, always rests its head or foot on his master and will not leave him.

◆ There are a lot of assistive technologies available now that will let you know where the person is, even within their house, and even if you can't see them or have gone out yourself. There has been bad publicity about these technologies from time to time, equating them with the 'tagging' of criminals and ignoring the fact that the restriction of human rights through deprivation of liberty is probably worse than a locator device.

Dot Gibson, NPC [National Pensioners Convention] general secretary, said, '... This is trying to solve a human problem with technology. Rather than tagging people we need better social care out in the community. Dementia patients need human interaction not tagging. Using electronic tags on dementia sufferers raises very important issues about the individual's human rights. They haven't committed any crime – they've just grown old. Older people are effectively being demonised and treated like criminals.'

Neil Duncan-Jordan, national officer of the National Pensioners Convention, called the practice 'inhumane' and said, 'It smacks of criminality' and puts them 'on a par with common offenders ... We should not be looking at dementia sufferers in that way.

'There has got to be a more humane way of coping with somebody's mental state, and, if it has got to that extreme level, it does beg the question: are there not proper facilities to care for people when they have severe cases of dementia?' (www.homecare.co.uk)

To be honest there is nothing very liberating about being locked in because you are likely to stray, or dying in a ditch because you got lost and no one could find you. However, these people have real concerns, which may be allayed when they consider that people in the early stages of dementia say that they value this assistive technology. It's not an alternative to care. It's an addition. Find out more about assistive technology in chapter 9 (page 226).

◆ Years ago there was a community that created an 'organised wandering' system. It was relatively rural and (with the right permissions) as many people as possible were informed about the two men in the area who were likely to go for a walkabout and not find their way back. Each day they'd be provided with the right footwear and clothes and be let loose. Of course there were risks, but the risks of attempting to deprive them of their liberty by restraining them at home were also significant. They included the likelihood of the men being sedated, with all the side effects involved, and the possibility of them getting aggressive with those who wanted to keep them in. People guided them back, or went walking with them. These days sophisticated tracking devices mean you'd always be able to find people, even if the community turned the other way and did not take care of them.

◆ You might have already had some narrow escapes. Part of your plan must be to make a list of the places where the person is likely to go. Your previous home, their favourite café ... you know that person's usual haunts. Research from search and rescue organisations emphasises that men and women have different wandering patterns. Men are more likely to go off the beaten track. Women are more likely to head for the shops. It sounds like a sexist cliché, but if it helps find them, who's complaining? If you have that horrible moment of panic when the person seems to have got lost, it is important that you are able to give the police or helpful neighbours the best possible description. Remembering what they were wearing is a good start, but a recent digital photo that can be quickly shared is useful. Take a new one frequently.

◆ Almost always the person is found. When that has happened, you have to relax. You are doing the best you can and you can't be criticised for it. Be careful not to make your home into a prison for yourself, because that is worse. You have established your plan for this happening again, and you will be even more efficient the next time. The Alzheimer's Foundation of America produced guidance in 2012 called 'Lost and Found', which is a review of methods and technologies for law enforcement agencies to help them locate missing adults with dementia. It includes advice on prevention, including environmental modification, and exit controls. It also lists 'Silver Alert Plans' in a number of states. It is more useful to know about these things before you actually need them. (www.alzfdn.org/documents/Lost&Found_forweb.pdf).

Other difficult things

When someone has dementia you may reach a stage where you are more involved than you ever expected to be with their bodily functions.

Incontinence is a bit of an issue but I've had two visits from the continence nurse and I've got a little routine sorted out. I treat him like a puppy. After each meal I take him to the toilet and sit him down and he usually does his business then. I only get soiled pants occasionally at night so the laundry isn't too awful. (Janice, wife of James, 81)

This gracious older lady is managing a difficult problem with an intensely practical and unemotional response. Incontinence is an issue that would cause people to have to go into care. Whatever you might think about the way she describes it, she's doing an amazing job and keeping her husband where he will be best loved and looked after – at home. There is no point in entering into discussion with her about privacy or dignity. In the quiet of their own home she has found a solution that creates the right balance for them and she knows what she is doing.

There are practical issues about how to wash faeces or solid waste off bedclothes or take it off other furniture. It is not pleasant to think about, but the most important thing is to scrape off excess solids into the toilet, and soak the bedding in a detergent that contains enzymes. Before washing in hot water, do what you can to get rid of faeces stains, because warm water can set the stain in. You can launder sheets in cool water with washing powder and colour-safe bleach. Be prepared by having cleaning gloves, disposable plastic bags and paper towels on hand, and the right detergent. There is a cheerful website called Housewife How-to's that has even more advice in this line. http://housewifehowtos.com/clean/how-to-clean-poop/.

As the American organisation, the National Association for Continence (NAC) says, 'Let's get past the embarrassment and on with our lives.' They report that over 25 million Americans are affected by incontinence, but that successes are on the rise. In their really useful website on www.nafc.org they recognise the fact that this is a really sensitive area, but they give practical advice.

For example, they talk about the smell of urine. Normal urine does not smell bad. Doctors used to diagnose diabetes from sweet smelling urine. If you are dehydrated or have an infection that is when trouble with bad smells arises and in addition some foods change the smell and look of pee. For example, red berries and beetroot can make it red, looking scarily like there is blood there. Blood in your urine is serious, so see a doctor if you've not been grazing on fresh red fruit and veg. Good juices for bladder health include cranberry and other non-citrus juices. If someone drips urine onto clothing, it will start to smell unpleasant after a while.

After voiding or having bowel movements, wipe from front to back. Clean the area after each pad or appliance change with a gentle cleanser — rinsing and drying thoroughly. If the skin is dry or reddened, a moisturizing cream may

*be used. For further skin protection, a protective ointment
(not urine soluble) may be applied to the skin as a final step.
(National Association for Continence)*

The NAC gives advice on urine collection devices and
adult briefs and pads. But it doesn't accept that incontinence is inevitable with aging and it recommends that
the person with dementia has a consultation with a
doctor or specialist nurse for advice. It could be that the
person has a medical problem that is treatable, or that
they are finding going to the toilet more complicated,
including locating it and getting out of their clothes in
time. There is more on this in chapters 9 and 12.

It is important to repeat and reinforce that people
need plenty to drink, particularly when they have
dementia. Commonly, after an embarrassing episode
of incontinence, older people restrict their fluid intake
to 'prevent accidents'. This course of action is likely to
give rise to an infection in the urinary system (UTI).
This can lead to two major problems. A UTI can make
a person with dementia increasingly confused, or can
cause confusion in a frail person who does not yet have
dementia. So the first problem is one where cognitive
problems get worse. The second problem is that the
infection makes the person need the toilet even more
often and more urgently than before, increasing the
chance of the 'accidents' they were trying to avoid.
A UTI is one of the common causes of a hospital
admission for people who until then were surviving
nicely at home. Keep the fluids going.

While many of us could contemplate discussing some of the intimate bodily issues that arise, there are some relationship issues that are so personal, so taboo, that it is almost impossible to enter into discussion with anyone. This may be particularly difficult for older people who have never been encouraged to talk much about relationships or sex.

He's stronger than me, and since this dementia set in, he's been a bit of a handful. He wants to go to bed with me three times a day for sex. It's as if he's forgotten about it immediately after. It is bad enough that he is so indiscreet about it, but these demands are too much. The nurse suggested distracting him but he gets aggressive if I refuse. (Eleanor, 79)

Changes in a couple's sex life are to be expected if one is ill and the other is exhausted with caring, but the behaviour described above is more akin to aggression and you would need professional help if it is a problem. Sexual hyperactivity is a concern that should be referred to the psychiatric service. Your safety and well-being should be the primary concern of your doctor, but it may be that you also need to talk to a counselling organisation if you find it really hard to open up about the subject. You must be reassured, though, that this problem is not unheard of and there may be medication that can help.

Another area that causes disturbance is something doctors call 'repetitive vocalisation'.

I need help with dealing with repeated questions. It was

suggested that I repeat the answer using the same words.
But what if it gets asked again and again? It's all too easy
to let the ... exasperation show. Sometimes I'd just end up
saying, 'Oh, you know, I've forgotten,' and Mum would
laugh (I'm not sure how comfortable a laugh that was
though). (Ruth, whose mother had dementia)

This repetitive behaviour is one of the most annoying
and intractable problems in dementia. No one knows
what to do about it, apart from distraction. For a
caregiver, being able to zone out is very good. Teenagers
often seem to know how to say 'Uh-huh' at the right
point in a conversation without actually being aware
of or paying attention to what is being said to them. If
we knew how they do that we could teach it to family
caregivers for selective use in times of desperation.

We know that disturbing behaviour in people with
dementia is often a response to their misunderstanding
and fear about what is happening to them. We can do a
lot to reduce that behaviour by removing or changing
the triggers. It is important to watch out for the way
in which health and social care staff may exacerbate
such behaviour. You might think that these are people
who should know better, but they may not have had
any education in this area. The care worker who is
accustomed to cheerfully and confidently walking
into a stranger's house, undressing them and diving
in and out of their rooms, moving and handling their
possessions, is just doing her job. She assumes that her
client has agreed to and even wants her services. But
if her client has dementia they may not remember

ever having agreed, so her 'normal' style is going to cause problems. If you have any control or influence at all, use it to indicate that you want staff to be not just 'dementia aware' but educated in how to manage dementia in a person's home. All your hard work should not be undone by people who are supposed to be helping.

Remember that what you are dealing with is very hard at times and make sure to give yourself a break.

chapter 8

Staying at home

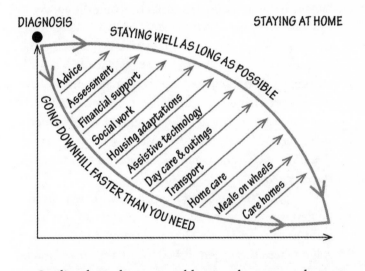

DIAGNOSIS · STAYING AT HOME

STAYING WELL AS LONG AS POSSIBLE

Advice
Assessment
Financial support
Social work
Housing adaptations
Assistive technology
Day care & outings
Transport
Home care
Meals on wheels
Care homes

GOING DOWNHILL FASTER THAN YOU NEED

Studies show that many older people want, and expect, to stay at home until they die, but they don't seriously prepare for it and don't do anything until circumstances force them to do so. They don't make preparations in their current home, and they have a narrow view of what help around the house they'd find acceptable in future.

Can you stay at home for ever? Most people with dementia live at home and half of those with dementia in the UK who live in their own home live alone. In other countries this varies. In the United States, it may be even higher, though this is hard to measure because so many have not been diagnosed, and so cannot be counted. In other countries, the number of people at home varies. For example, in countries where there is not a highly developed care home or nursing home industry, like India, nearly everyone with dementia is currently living at home. In countries with access to low cost overseas domestic staff, such as Hong Kong or Singapore, it is possible to stay at home with such support for longer. Change is taking place as women's working patterns and the numbers of children they have to support change, and that is why having dementia and staying at home is often described as a 'women's issue'. In the USA almost two thirds of people with dementia are women, and they make up two thirds of the caregivers.

It is perfectly possible for a person with dementia to be happy at home for a long time and to do very well, right to the end of life. However, some people reach a stage where they need to be looked after more intensively. Dementia is a long-term condition that gradually worsens, but many people with dementia become ill and die of something else before the symptoms get too serious, so it's important to plan for living well and not feel that everything has suddenly shuddered to a halt the day the diagnosis is given. This chapter gives some help in understanding how to make care at home work.

My dad started to lose some of his words and reached

the point where he could not spell his own name. But we
travelled and walked and worked in the garden right up
till the day he had his heart attack and died. (Daughter of
67-year-old man with early-onset dementia)

In general people want to put off as long as possible the
time when they might have to give up their own home
to go to other accommodation. Good care homes and
nursing homes are in despair because of bad publicity
about a small number of really unsatisfactory care
homes. The good ones provide charming and comfortable places for people to live in at a difficult time of
life; but calamitous stories dominate the press and
public imagination. A 2013 newscast from CTV news
in Canada is typical of the sort of story that worries
people. It reported suspension of staff after secret
filming in a care home:

After the release of shocking video of an elderly woman
with dementia being subjected to abuse and humiliation at
a southern Ontario long-term care facility, many are saying
the incident is far from isolated ... Montreal-based lawyer
Jean-Pierre Menard has handled countless cases of abuse
at nursing homes and long-term care facilities including a
horrific case against the St-Charles Borromée hospital in
*Montreal. (*http://www.ctvnews.ca/canada/nursing-home-
abuse-incident-not-isolated-say-experts-1.1290010*)*

This kind of reporting shapes the perception of families
and friends when they are considering moving someone
into a care home. Many people at the early stages of
dementia are quite adamant that they want to stay at

home for ever. Some even say that they'd rather have euthanasia than go into care. We all love our homes. You spend your whole life getting it just the way you want it, so why would you leave it and go somewhere else, particularly when you're not feeling right? In this chapter there are ideas about how to stay at home for as long as possible. But there is a postscript reminding you that if you do move to a care home or nursing home it is not a sign of failure or betrayal. A day may come when you think it is right for such a move. You can be kind to your family by telling them that when the day comes, even if you are not well enough to take part in the decision, you accept that this is what they may have to do for you. You need to trust someone else to do what is best for you and that is why choosing the right person to have power of attorney is so important (see Chapter 13).

In the beginning: preparation and enjoying life to the full

Getting used to the idea of what dementia really means takes time. It is possible that there has been a lot of worry about what was going wrong and at least now you have a name to put to it. If you've had experience of someone with dementia in the family before, it is worth getting up-to-date information because a lot has changed in recent years.

My grandmother had it, and there were no pills, and it was the sort of thing you kept secret. They just said 'she's senile' and we all looked the other way until it fell apart in her house and we got her into hospital. Then she went in a home. (Andrew, 55)

In all developed countries, health department policies are driving doctors to make a diagnosis earlier and earlier. This means that, hopefully, when you learn that dementia is the problem there will still be a whole lot of living to do before life gets really tough. This is precious time during which you can enjoy your home and your home life. If the person with dementia does not live with you, there are things that you can do together to make preparation for the future. If you are affected by dementia yourself, you can do things to keep yourself well and happy for as long as possible.

Advance preparations

You may be wondering about whether to move home. In general staying put is the best idea for people with dementia. Moving to a new location can be harrowing for any of us. It takes a lot of planning and physical energy and there is the worry about mortgages, tenancy agreements or leases, how much it costs and whether it is the right thing to do. If the motivation is something wonderful like a new garden, more space or a new job it can be brilliant. However, if you are not feeling well and the move is not for a positive reason, it could be traumatic, especially if it feels like putting one foot in the grave. A person with dementia might feel coerced into it.

I want Dad to move to be near us because he is getting dementia and I want to look after him. He wants to stay put but that's not an option. I've told him and he's not happy. (Mrs B., 60, daughter with power of attorney for her father)

Nevertheless, not everyone wants to stay on their own. If you have been widowed, and live by yourself, you may feel lonely and isolated. You could decide to move nearer family, whether that is in their home, in nearby special housing where you can get assistance, or just in another house or apartment nearby. If you are going to have to move there are design issues about the new place which you should consider (see Chapter 9) and it is best to make the move while you are feeling physically healthy. If it is inevitable, then it's best to move in a controlled way, rather than as a result of an emergency.

Davinia had a fall at home and went into hospital, so I gave up the house and when she came out I moved her straight into the new place. (Nephew of a woman with dementia)

Everything works better when we feel we have some choice and control, and this is especially true for a person with dementia. It's important to minimise the number of moves that a person with dementia has to make, because increasing stress often makes dementia symptoms worse. Having to learn a new environment is particularly difficult. Planning is really important, to iron out as many details of the move as possible in advance.

There is a clear and growing need for services which

are available shortly after diagnosis and which focus expressly on helping someone to carry on living independently in their own home. There are lots of models of this so the main issue is whether there is one near you. The best way to find these now is via the Internet. There is such a complex web of organisations and what they offer is so diverse and changing that there is no book that can link you to a local organisation efficiently. Some of the Internet links are, however, listed at the end of this book.

One of the determining factors will be finance. In Scotland there is a government guarantee of one year's post-diagnostic support from the health and social care system, focused on information about your options and 'signposting'. This is unusual. Some voluntary organisations will do a 'wealth check' for you to help you work out whether you are getting all the financial assistance to which you are entitled. If there is no non-profit near you that can do this, it is worth talking to an independent financial adviser about how to manage the cost of your future care needs. It is never too soon to get started with this. Staying at home is made possible by a range of interventions, some of which cost a lot of money. People in Australia, Canada and the UK are fortunate in the extent to which there is a safety net for people who don't have savings, but even there dementia care is much more expensive than cancer or other conditions because a lot of the care is defined as 'social care' rather than 'health care' and is therefore means tested in a different way. This is a good time to talk to your chosen welfare attorney about what you want for the future and what you have covered. They will have to decide on your behalf if you can't do so later because of illness, but you need to make sure that they understand your thinking while you are still able to tell them.

What are the options for housing support or supported housing?

Housing design and supported housing organisations will pay an increasingly important role in improving the world for people with dementia. Delaying the need for residential care is a major part of controlling the financial burden. If the home setting is good, it could shorten the length of a hospital stay, allowing the person to return home quickly, and helping to prevent them having to go from hospital to a care home. There are many examples of good practice from housing associations and home improvement agencies that provide specialist housing, adaptations for your own house and a range of flexible support:

Over the next ten years, the number of people [in England] living with dementia is set to rise to over one million. The majority of these people will live in the community, in their own homes, and they want to stay there for as long as possible. Early intervention services centred on people's homes have the greatest potential to improve the quality of life of people with dementia and their carers. (Alistair Burns, National Clinical Director for Dementia for England)

The concept of a tailored design of house or apartment for a person with dementia has been around since the 1980s. This not only concerns the design of the residence and the use of assistive technology, but also embraces the idea of staff who are trained to come and give support to you in that setting, while allowing you to live independently for as long as possible. When looking for this sort of place you will find it called 'housing with care', 'extra care housing', 'assisted living' and 'continuing-care housing'. Special training courses are available for staff at these facilities, specifically on supporting people with dementia at home.

The US Department of Housing and Urban Development (HUD) provides a public housing programme. Public housing aims to provide decent and safe rental housing for eligible low-income families, older people, and people with disabilities. The HUD administers Federal aid to local housing agencies (HAs) that manage the housing for low-income residents. Long waiting periods are common, but each HA has the discretion to establish preferences to reflect the needs in its own community and in some places that includes old age and frailty including dementia. It is means tested. A local organisation may advertise HUD subsidised apartments, including the offer of personal care.

For 60 years Wesley Woods has been making the retirement experience healthy and fulfilling for older adults of all income levels, races, and faiths. Throughout Atlanta and across North Georgia, we operate comfortable retirement communities that emphasize wellness, socialization, education, and personal and spiritual fulfillment for our residents. Several retirement communities have levels of care that allow residents to 'transition in place' as their needs change. As a not-for-profit provider, Wesley Woods provides affordable residential and healthcare services to older adults. This support makes Wesley Woods different from the many profit-based retirement communities that are rapidly being built in our community, because at Wesley Woods we serve people rather than the bottom line. (information from a Christian Methodist housing organisation that serves all income levels including those who have outlived their resources).

Through its faith based mission, Wesley Woods 'strives to help people age with grace'. How to find something like this in your own area or country, if you need it, will vary, and also how to find a secular organisation, or one from your own faith base. For people in the United States and Canada 'A Place for Mom' www.aplaceformom. com/ provides advice to help families navigate the maze of housing options for seniors. It has grown to become the largest senior living referral service. It is paid for by the participating communities and providers in their network, so advice is offered at no charge to families.

These housing schemes can be designed for generalised groups of retired people, so sometimes the management or the other residents are not very tolerant of people with dementia. In many cases they are operated by non-profit housing associations, but businesses are also seizing opportunities to serve the dementia market.

Retirement villages and complexes

A retirement village was traditionally a housing complex designed for older people who care for themselves, but increasingly these complexes have other levels of supported accommodation to which the residents can move when their needs rise over time. The idea of owning a place in a private retirement village may appeal to those who have the means to buy the apartment, studio flat or house and pay the maintenance or service charges. This typically would offer the comfort of a luxury high-specification cottage or apartment and a range of facilities in a secluded environment. People can move into the community when they are over the age of fifty-five and undergo transition to an onsite care home if that is subsequently required. In the USA they might have 100,000 residents. The European versions are more modest in size. You may prefer to live in a smaller complex, which could be a block of retirement flats or a small scheme of ground-level houses in a mixed area such as a real town or village, so that you see and meet people of different ages and can access facilities that everyone else uses.

Although the [retirement] village looked great, we really needed to have a think about all the questions. Could I bring my own furniture and was my dog allowed to come? Was there any control over the service charges? It turned out that there was something called an 'assignment fee' that I had to consider. I needed to get my lawyer to advise me. Then it turned out that they wanted a report from my doctor as well that I was in 'good health'. I decided against that one. (M., 72)

Funding such a move may be prohibitive for many. You need independent legal and financial advice for all of this.

In the United States and Canada, the websites of care complexes offer advice on financial packages. Their advisers 'help seniors and family members navigate through the many options available to finance assisted living' as one brochure puts it. These options can include an unsecured line of credit, or secured lending options such as a home loan. In the United States they also work with Veterans Administration staff to help you apply for assisted living benefits, if you are eligible, including Aid and Attendance. A life insurance policy could be converted into a long-term care benefit. So you definitely need legal and independent financial advice. This kind of advice is sometimes available at discounted rates through membership of an organisation, such as AARP. Advice is available free through an annual initiative called Financial Planning Days in twenty-five cities in the United States, but you always have to check the credentials of the person giving advice. A good place to start is www.letsmakeaplan.org.

The Australian Government has established a service called My Aged Care http://www.myagedcare.gov.au/ It is part of the Australian Government's changes to the aged care system which have been designed to give people more choice, more control and easier access to a full range of aged care services. It is made up of a website and a contact centre giving information on aged care for yourself, a family member, friend or someone you're caring for. It provides help to find Government-funded aged care services. 'Sorted – the Kiwi guide to money' https://www.sorted.org.nz/life-events/moving-to-a-retirement-village offers checklists of the sort of questions that a New Zealander might ask before making a commitment.

Living with relatives

Living with relatives can be wonderful. A multigenerational family can have lots of fun. Of course there are areas of stress too, as when any family members choose to live together. If young people move back home to live with parents, rules and boundaries can be set to avoid conflicts, but for a person with dementia, a condition that changes, it is sometimes difficult to make hard and fast rules.

However, there are some simple strategies that you can adopt – for example, having certain rooms, such as the bedroom, that are private, and knocking before entering. If you've taken in a parent or moved in with them, don't take all their chores and activities from them. Keeping on doing things is good for a person with dementia. You need to be clear about compensation and what the financial arrangements will be. That is simpler if you have power of attorney, but even so, it's a good idea to keep the rest of the family informed about what is happening in case of misunderstandings. If you set goals and clearly communicate plans it will prevent some potential battles.

You might want to consider what you'd do if the family situation broke down.

Sally and Harry were married for three years when Harry's grandmother Bertha moved in with them. Bertha, who had early signs of dementia, was struggling in the community. Things were fine till Sally and Harry's marriage started to fail two years later because of Harry's infidelity. Sally had paid for most of the house by working overseas a lot, but Harry wanted to keep the house because he needed it as principal carer for his grandmother. He could not afford to buy out his share of their home. Bertha was suddenly not sure about where she was going to live. (from Dementia: the One-Stop Guide)

Sometimes, though, it is a happy situation and a great blessing for young and old.

My mother moved in with us, and this is the best move we ever made. She loves the children and they can spend so much time with her. When she shuts the door on her part of the house at night, she is completely private, but she could call us if she needed us. She's in the early stage of dementia and we know we might have to rethink one day, but we are fine at present. (Janice, daughter of M., 72)

Perhaps you could stay where you are. If you've lived there for a long time, lapses in recent memory are not so serious, because you'd still find your way home.

The situation is different in different countries. People in countries like New Zealand and the UK, which have traditionally expected elder care to be provided by the government, sometimes have a suspicion about the for-profit age care sector, perhaps considering that the low wages of staff is allowing the owners to line their own pockets with money. But in places where families have to pay directly themselves for care, the family will try to keep the cost down as much as any commercial provider does. Employing 'maids' or foreign domestic workers is a transnational multi-million dollar industry that provides a lot of dementia care in Hong Kong and Singapore, and works out cheaper for the family and the state than putting someone in a care home. Having a foreign domestic worker is so common in Singapore that the local Alzheimer's Disease Association provides training programmes for maids:

'Caring for A Person With Dementia' is a training workshop comprising of seven elective modules, the modular training will be conducted from 9.00am to 12.30pm and 1.30pm to 4.30pm at our ADA Resource & Training Centre. It is open strictly for FDWs [Foreign Domestic Workers] caring for people with dementia. You may register online any of the seven modules here. (Advertisement on the ADA website) http://www.alz.org.sg/

Kirsten Han, a Singaporean journalist, has written about this 'strange mix of opportunity and exploitation'. When it was made compulsory in 2013 that the maids should have a paid day off, there was a backlash from employers. The work of one-to-one care of a person with dementia in the family home seems tough to some observers, though some maids are very happy and send much needed money to their families at home. And at least the person with dementia is able to continue being looked after at home, and not institutionalised. Though having live-in help is not affordable for most people, it highlights the research that demonstrates that dementia care is fundamentally women's work. Where there is a supply of women who are prepared to care for no wages in their own family, or for low wages in someone else's family or country, this can work out less expensive and more comfortable to the person with dementia than alternatives. Families do not hesitate to manage the need for care in this way. In every country of the world, the health and social care system is dependent on the unpaid care provided by families at home for people with dementia. This is true even where it is assumed that there is a well-funded health and social care system.

Local authority or housing association supported sheltered housing

Many local authorities in the UK run sheltered housing, mainly one-bedroom homes, which are adapted for people with particular needs or disabilities. The houses might have a built-in alarm system, including monitoring of activity in many cases. Some have community rooms, laundry facilities or guest rooms for use by families. In some cases meals are also provided and that is sometimes called 'very sheltered housing'. In addition to the weekly rent for your house, you will probably pay a service charge, which covers the cost of the alarm system and responses and any agreed-upon housing support. A housing support officer is usually available to help you complete any forms, in particular if you have a low income and are eligible for housing benefit. When you move in, a support worker is allocated to you and they assess what support you will need. This could include help to attend appointments or social activities, and help with managing your mail or paying bills.

In the United States there is increasing recognition that housing for older people needs to be in a community setting that provides a range of services, but particularly health care. The AARP Foundation has been supporting Leading Age (www.leadingage.org) a membership organisation of 6,000 non-profit organisations, in creating a Housing Plus Services guide based on the best practices of twelve providers who are called the Housing Plus Services Collaborative.

The number of older Canadians is increasing, and because some are now continuing to work after the age of sixty-five, it makes it less attractive for them to move to a retirement community. Many older Canadians have access to pensions, private and public, and many own their own homes.

Canada has many older people who immigrated to the country, and their support needs are different depending on when they migrated and their ethnic origin. About 80 per cent of Canadians live in urban areas, and urban seniors are more likely to experience social isolation, indicating that physical isolation is not the only cause of loneliness. First Nations communities have particular needs and the resources available to them are outlined in the Indiginous and Northern

Affairs Canada Website; www.aadnc-aandc.gc.ca. For other useful foundations please see Helpful Organisations section p. 355.

Rest, respite and home care

Day care services can help to maintain someone at home. The private sector also has a long tradition of offering these services. If money is no object you can have all of them, but even if you are reliant on health care and social care, many services could be available if they assess you as needing them and they have the resources in your local area.

◆ Complex care services can be provided at home when someone has been discharged from hospital and has significant nursing care needs that require continuous monitoring.

◆ Night care is available where an agency provides a nurse, careworker or support worker to support sleeping and to deal with any disturbances or care needs in the night. They can help with bathing and getting someone ready for bed, and they will provide drinks. They can even wear night-time clothes to help avoid confusion when the person wakes up. The night-time person can arrange to be awake all the time, or retire to sleep and be on call when you need them.

◆ When the person with dementia approaches the end of life, there is a great temptation to transfer them to hospital even though health care professionals could provide care round the clock at home.

◆ Vacation care can be provided in the person's own home so that the caregiver can go away. Some agencies will even offer a hotel call out service, so that you could get help at your holiday location if you go away together.

◆ Live-in care is available from agencies for varying lengths of time, not just vacation respite.

◆ Hospital to home services can support a person who wants to go back home after a hospital admission. Many people with dementia end up staying in hospital after their medical needs have passed, because there is no one to help with that transition.

◆ Help with household activities, the daily routine, day trips out and social activities can be what enables someone to stay at home. Families can do a lot, but in their absence voluntary organisations and other friends can be invaluable.

In Washington DC there is a membership group that is designed to support elders to stay at home in their neighbourhoods. Called Senior Villages, they facilitate access to community support services and connection to the life of the community. They are grassroots membership-based organisations, and they offer cultural and health activities as well as member-to-member volunteer support. They say,

*The need for this is clear; research shows that the most damaging threat to well being in later life is not fear of absolute destitution or poor health but loss of life purpose and boredom. (*www.dcoa.gov/service/senior-villages*)*

It's important to remember that the majority of people with dementia stay at home in the last weeks of their lives, and this is achievable, even if it takes a bit of organizing. There is a high likelihood that any one of us will have difficulty in arranging to die in our own bed at home. Many people get rushed to hospital at the end – at times without any real benefit. Advance directives and other mechanisms described in Chapter 13 will give you some idea of how to avoid that, if you want to think about it at all.

chapter 9

Your dementia-friendly home

By 'home' I mean the house or apartment where you live. This can be a place that you've lived in for a long time, or somewhere you've moved to in later years, or perhaps you have moved very recently to help deal with practical problems associated with dementia. Some of the ideas in this chapter are about changes that you can make now and others are things you could consider if you were moving to a new or purpose-built place. There are suggestions that are inexpensive and some that are fairly major, and you would not always do everything described here. For example, you would not change all the floor coverings in your house on the basis of this advice, but if you had decided to change them anyway you might consider these ideas when choosing your new flooring:

My husband is a cabinetmaker and builder and although neither of us has dementia or anything like it, we make dementia-friendly decisions whenever we are making any change in our house. It all looks really nice, not like some of the ugly adaptations that you see. So even if he passes away before me, and I get dementia, he'll have made sure that I can stay in our house for longer. (Mrs C., 62)

If you or someone who lives with you has dementia you've got a lot on your plate. Some of the problems that occur every day can't be avoided, but some of them can. If you sort out the avoidable problems by making adjustments in your home, you can concentrate your energies on the issues that are more difficult to resolve. Architects call this 'universal design' or 'design for life'.

General hints

◆ Remember that the person with dementia has difficulties with recall, working things out, learning new things and coping with disabilities or impairments, all of which is very stressful, so when you make any changes keep this in mind. It is fortunate if the person can stay in a familiar place for as long as possible. After a move they may wake up in the morning, having forgotten that they've moved, and try to get back to the old place. In some cases the dementia only really surfaces after a move. This demonstrates that an unfamiliar environment can challenge someone who is having problems with working things out, learning new things and remembering.

◆ In the person's own home change as little as possible apart from increasing the light and removing hazards. Even if you agree to throw out the old sofa, you'll be asked the next day where it is. The only changes you should make are those which are really required for safety and security. Decluttering is good if you can get away with it, but be aware that the person may turn round and ask for the object today that they asked you to throw away yesterday.

◆ If the person is moving to a new home, that is a chance to make things dementia-friendly. To be dementia-friendly everything should be 'obvious' – that is, it should be traditional in design and consistent with the person's culture and so make the place as stress-free as possible.

Light

Physiological changes in the eye mean that the capacity to see steadily deteriorates from a young age. By the time people are about 75 years old they need twice as much light as normal lighting standards recommend, and nearly four times as much as a 20-year-old, in order to see satisfactorily. The two implications … are that twice the 'normal' light is required, and that the lighting level in spaces should be set by someone who is of mature years. (Dementia Services Development Centre, 'Light and Lighting Design for People with Dementia')

◆ People with dementia are usually older. The lens, the clear part of the front of the eye, yellows over time, so it is as if the older person sees the world through a pair of yellow goggles that get thicker each year. Every old person needs to have more light to counteract this, but it is even more important in dementia. For example, if it is hard to remember where anything has been put, having lots of light means you can perhaps see it.

◆ Older eyes find it harder to adjust to changes in light levels, so if you have lights that switch on automatically with movement sensors, make sure that they go on earlier and stay on for longer. When I'm headed up the stairs, it's no use if the light does not go on until I am at the first step, because I will be halfway up before my eyes have adjusted to the new light level. Watch out if the optician is trying to persuade your dad to have a photo-chromic tint on his bifocals. It is all very well trying to look like a Mafioso with shades on, but he might fall over when he steps back into the house from the sunlight.

◆ Energy-saving light bulbs will make a contribution to saving the planet, but if your dad was an early adopter of that technology he probably bought his a number of years ago, when they still had a problem with longevity. The newer light bulbs seem to shine brightly compared with first wave ones which year on year lose their luminosity.

We've got some of those energy-saving bulbs in our house that seem to suck light in rather than give any out. You'd need a miner's lamp to light your way about. (C., daughter of Mr C., 63)

◆ The cheapest light comes through the windows. Get curtain rods that allow the curtains to open right back to maximise the aperture. If the window faces a wall, paint the wall white to reflect light back in. Cut back outside vegetation and clean the glass. Beware of glare, but there are ways of reducing that without reducing light: for example, using fine netting. Netting also helps with the problem of windows behaving like mirrors at night. If the person sees their own reflection in the glass when it is dark, they might misinterpret what they see. Have the electric lights on all the time, with light sensors that just switch them off when the natural light reaches the required level.

◆ Daylight has the added advantage that it helps to set the body clock, the internal mechanism that makes you sleepy at night. Melatonin is the naturally occurring hormone that sets your body clock. International travellers buy it in pill form to help them overcome jet lag. In your body the production of this useful molecule is reduced in old age and even further in dementia. It's one of the reasons that people with dementia turn night into day. Its metabolism is stimulated by daylight falling on the retina at the back of the eye, particularly the spectrum of light in the early part of the day. Getting out in daylight can make it more likely that the person will sleep (there is more on this in the section about bedrooms: see page 231).

◆ If you are going to change one thing only, increase the wattage of the light bulbs throughout the house. Avoid subtle or subdued lighting. More is better, but you must check the maximum wattage of the light fixtures to make sure they are not being overloaded. If there is a pendant light in the room with three bulbs, replace it with one with five. The more, the better.

◆ Some of the useful objects in the house need to be

more obvious than before. If the person always had a bedside clock, get a bigger one and put it in exactly the same place. Make sure that their glasses prescriptions are up to date. Optometrists will come and see you at home very happily in some countries, for example the UK. Such services are starting to appear in the United States. In their offices optometrists have equipment that will test for a range of eye problems and can often refer you directly to the eye hospital if there is a serious problem.

I dreaded her getting cataracts done when the optician said my mum needed it. Our grandmother had to lie still in hospital for days after when she had it. But it is quick these days. It took about half an hour and we had to be careful for a day or two, but it got better really fast. It has given her a new lease of life. She started watching her movies again and keeping herself occupied happily in the day. She was getting miserable before. (Daughter of D., 92)

Sound

Losing your hearing is a bit like going to a foreign country where you speak only a bit of the language. You struggle ... and just trying to get by leaves you exhausted. This is exactly what happens to people who suffer hearing loss. As a result, they may start to withdraw from many of the activities they used to enjoy, because certain scenarios might tire them out, or might be embarrassing or difficult. Now we think this could have a worrying knock-on effect: evidence is emerging that deafness may lead to dementia ...

Whether one is causing the other, or whether they're simply associated, is not clear. But we do know that deafness leads to a greater cognitive load. And if your brain has to make more of an effort to do one task, it will be compromised in others. (Professor David McAlpine, Director of the University College London Ear Institute, Mail Online, 12 March 2013)

◆ If you have good concentration you can ignore what is going on around you. When concentration is difficult, extraneous noise makes life difficult, particularly if you are prone to misinterpreting noises because of cognitive impairment. Take time to sit in your house with your eyes closed and listen to the noises round about. See what you can do to reduce any of them.

◆ Remember the difference between sound and noise. After they get a hearing aid, people tell you that it's difficult at first. Everything is amplified, so the noise of, say, the air conditioning and traffic is as noticeable as the sound of voices in the room. They have a problem in differentiating between background noise and meaningful sounds. People with dementia seem to have a similar difficulty. It's hard for anyone to concentrate if there are lots of distracting noises and they are tired. Anything you can do in your house to minimise meaningless noise is valuable. If you have an impaired capacity to think, you need all the help you can get.

◆ Having the TV or radio on when no one is watching or listening is an obvious issue. It makes life difficult for the person with dementia. Music can help people to relax and that works best if it is their favourite music, so an iPod with personalised music tracks is ideal. It's better than listening to the radio, where music is often interrupted with commercial breaks, news or pointless chatter. Design the auditory environment so that you can get positive benefits from what the person can hear and eliminate the negative effect of communal undifferentiated noise.

A movie has been made to document the 'Music & Memory' project ... familiar music from our youth is often untouched during the course of the disease. No matter the degree of memory loss, music has the power to help us feel whole, lift our mood, reduce anxiety, and help us feel more alive. Alive Inside: A Story of Music and Memory *follows Dan Cohen, a social worker who decides on a whim to bring iPods to a nursing home. What Dan Cohen discovers by accident, and scientists have been studying for years, is that a person suffering from memory loss can seem to 'awaken' when given music they have an emotional attachment to. As Oliver Sacks explains, 'Music imprints itself on the brain deeper than any other human experience. Music evokes emotion and emotion can bring with it memory.' (Reported by Alzheimer's Disease International)*

◆ Soft furnishings like carpets and curtains help to absorb noise. The current fashion for wood-effect flooring is very practical and hygienic, but carpet tiles can give a high level of hygiene while reducing the clatter that comes from furniture scraping about and the noise of feet.

◆ Make sure that hearing aids are well maintained and that more than one person knows how to adjust them and replace the batteries. Controls can be very small and awkward. Remember that a build-up of earwax can occur at any time and get ears checked regularly. You must not assume that the person does not understand you because of their dementia when in fact they are just not hearing you because they need a nurse to syringe their ears.

◆ Studies show that people do not get themselves a hearing aid until years after they would benefit, so consider a test. People who lack their back teeth seem to risk a build-up of excess impacted earwax because its production and elimination are promoted by jaw movement. The local nurse will be able to syringe ears regularly if the doctor can see that sort of problem, which is increased by the use of hearing aids because they cause the wax to become impacted.

In medieval times they used earwax for the preparation of pigments for illuminated manuscripts. Now the doctor usually doesn't even check after syringing to see if it has been removed. It's worth asking for them to do that even if you are not going to make personal use of it. (Dementia nurse)

Floor coverings

◆ There is evidence that a person with dementia will walk more swiftly and safely over a smooth, matte, un-patterned surface. Being able to move about depends on a whole range of factors, including how fit you are, how mobile, what shoes you have on and whether you can see. Having the floor covering right is just one element. However, if being slow to get moving makes the difference between getting to the bathroom in time and not, you can see the benefit in having the right flooring. Avoid patterns. No shiny walking surfaces. Have the floor contrast with the walls and try to use the same colour throughout to avoid 'junctions' where one room colour meets another, which is made particularly difficult if there is an obvious threshold strip.

The interior designers for the new hospital fancied a floor pattern that divided the corridor flooring along the full length with two-thirds being darker than the other third – two shades of grey. We said that this would not be 'dementia-friendly' due to depth-perception problems. They ignored this. Now the nurses tell us that old people are falling over in those areas. (Dementia Services Development Centre [DSDC] design team leader)

◆ The changes in how well a person with dementia walks may be caused by the underlying disease, which leads to coordination difficulties in some cases. All of us stumble once in a while, but the danger with dementia or simple frailty is being slow to recover from a stumble and consequently falling. Trip hazards in the home may be really obvious and need to be dealt with as a matter of urgency. The community occupational therapist may be able to help with this, but mostly it is common sense. Imagine shuffling through the house, then check what would trip you, including door thresholds and little mats.

◆ Any hard surfaces, such as ramps indoors and out, and bathroom and kitchen floors, should be covered with one of the commercial non-slip floor coverings that are available. These should reduce the likelihood of a fall even if wet.

◆ The flooring usually stops at a skirting board/baseboard where it meets the wall. Paint these boards a contrasting colour to the floor. Some people with depth-perception problems have difficulty in working out where this junction is, and this makes it hard to judge where they are putting their feet. For example, there is a fashion for taking the floor covering up the wall a few centimetres, which you often see in wet-rooms, mudrooms or shower rooms. It helps prevent water leaking, but unfortunately may create a visual illusion that the floor is a few centimetres or an inch higher than it really is and the consequent misplacing of a foot when the person tries to step up on entering the room can cause them to stumble.

◆ Much is made of colour coding in dementia and that is a real irritation for dementia experts because it does not help. Learning the meaning of a colour code is like learning a new language. That's not easy at this time. The most important thing to say about floor coverings is that they should contrast with the walls.

Decoration and furniture

◆ If you are considering redecorating the place where someone has lived for a long time, ask yourself why. It could be that the resulting turmoil makes it not worthwhile. Remember that just increasing the light is really helpful and much less effort.

◆ For the training of health and social care staff (and interior designers!) one can buy glasses that mimic a range of visual impairments, including those that are more common in older people with dementia. You want to check the environment? By wearing sunglasses smeared with petroleum jelly while trying to walk around the house, you can test the environment yourself for colour contrast, including noting the visibility of furniture, bedding and towels.

Contrast is the key to vision. If there is no contrast, objects cannot easily be seen and differentiated ... As we age we lose the ability to differentiate colours clearly, our perception of depth diminishes, there is a loss of visual acuity, we have less spatial awareness and our sensitivity to contrast lowers. Without good contrasts, the world becomes hazier, we struggle more and more to make sense of it and we function in life with less confidence. (DSDC Design Resource Centre)

◆ If you are wallpapering or painting, note that wall coverings with strong patterns can cause optical illusions for some people with dementia. Keep things simple, with bland colours for most walls and a high degree of contrast between the colours of doors, skirting and base boards and floors.

◆ Use light paint on the ceiling and hang light-coloured curtains. Particularly after dark, the curtains and ceiling take up a lot of the field of vision, so make use of the chance to reflect light into the room from them.

◆ I'm often asked about good and bad colours, and if they affect mood. There is no research evidence for mood alteration from colour in itself. However, someone like me might like Wedgwood blue specifically because it reminds me of the walls in my childhood home. In this way colour might help someone feel calm, safe and at home. It's not an intrinsic quality of the particular shade of blue that matters but the association. It is really hard to generalise.

◆ There is debate about whether there is good or bad art for people with dementia. Again, this is a question of taste and association. As recent memories fade, the collection of graduation photos of my grandchildren might start to lose meaning, but a youthful photo of my own mother may mean a lot to me right until I die. Some care homes go overboard with pictures of the local area in 'times gone by'. With the age range of residents being quite variable, and social and geographical mobility, this is often just a gimmick. It is nice and interesting, but it is not really related specifically to dementia care.

◆ If you are inclined to forget where useful objects are, glass-fronted cupboards and wardrobes are available and chests of drawers with open fronts to let you see what is inside. Of course you could also label the drawers.

◆ Mirrors (and other reflective surfaces) cause practical problems. If you have forgotten the last twenty years and you see an eighty-year-old version of yourself in the mirror, you will be inclined to think that it's not you. You are expecting to see a much younger person. You may think that this is a stranger looking through a window. You can cover mirrors and pull drapes over reflective window surfaces to prevent this disconcerting experience.

My mother had become incontinent and demonstrated agitated behaviour when we attempted to escort her to her ensuite shower room to use the toilet. She screamed and shouted and appeared to be saying that there was a 'devil' in there. We removed the mirror above the sink and she started to use the toilet normally again. (family member)

Assistive technology

There is a wide range of technological solutions to some of the common problems that living at home with dementia brings. Some of these solutions have been mentioned elsewhere in the book. This technology can be used for safety, for locating people who might get lost, for entertainment and for distraction. New products continue to be developed all the time, so it is important to keep an eye out for the latest products. Prices come down all the time and your local authority may be prepared to bear some of the cost as part of their effort to keep people living in the community. Check out the extremely valuable website www. atdementia.org.uk for ideas and prices.

At present in some countries no single private insurance plan or public programme that I am aware of gives comprehensive coverage for assistive technology (AT). It may be that in the United States Medicare, Medicaid or the Department of Veterans Affairs will pay for some. Most states in the US have an agency that deals with AT issues. Some Area Agencies on Aging have programmes that help people to access low cost AT, but searching national public websites shows few products that are specifically listed for cognitive impairment. It is worth browsing the AT Dementia website and using that as a springboard to find how you can access a particular product where you live. It will be there. The trick is finding what there is and how it might help. A good start would be the website www.atdementia.org.uk or the free download from DSDC at www.dementiashop.co.uk.

◆ If you are anxious about the person leaving the house and getting lost, consider a locator device that can be worn as a discreet wristband like a watch. There are many commercial brands available which include a facility to track your loved one by PC or smartphone. This has the advantage that you can allow or even encourage the person to go out and about, secure in the knowledge that you will be able to locate them if needed.

◆ Security of the home is an issue. The person may

leave the house without locking it or lose keys. They may be anxious about too many keys circulating in the community: for example, if there are careworkers in and out of the house from time to time. A key safe is a small box fixed to the wall or the door handle in which a spare key can be stored and accessed only by using a secret number. This means that legitimate visitors or carers can enter without anyone having to come to open the door, and the person does not need to answer the door if there is an unexpected or nuisance caller. Biometric locks are also commercially available and can store up to eighty fingerprints. This means that someone can open the door at a touch if they've been included on the list. The additional provision of an ordinary key and a combination lock makes secure access and door opening flexible for unexpected emergencies. It adds to safety because it locks automatically when the door is slammed shut, but can be opened from inside without a key at any time.

◆ Infrared emitters are useful, light and easy to install. They produce a beam which, when it is broken, can control room lights when the person enters or leaves an area. They can also be used to warn the caregiver that the person is on the move. This can be via a buzzer under a sleeping caregiver's pillow or a signal on their cellphone. You can also acquire an electronic monitoring system which involves very small wireless sensors being placed in the kitchen, bathroom, living room and bedroom to monitor the movement of

the person around their house. A family member
or caregiver can access this information via the
Internet and reassure themselves that the person with
dementia is up and about and doing normal things.
(www.justchecking.co.uk)

*I can log on to my laptop and see a chart of my dad's
movements about the house. It showed him always to be
getting up very early, so we arranged for home care before
six a.m. To begin with he thought we were going to be
filming him, but he now understands that there is no
camera or sound, just a blip on a screen when movement
happens in the room and that I don't look all the time, just a
couple of times each day or when I think of it. One brilliant
example is when the early-morning careworker wondered if
he was sleeping in the chair at night and not going to bed.
The movement monitor proved he was going to bed. He just
made the bed so neatly that it looked like it had not been
slept in. (Andrew, talking about Douglas, 92)*

◆ For people with dementia there is a problem when
relatives and the authorities are too risk-averse. People
forget that a person with dementia does have a right
to do unwise things. Electronic monitoring actually
helps give freedom to people with dementia because
it reassures the relatives. Over-anxious relatives have
in the past unnecessarily accelerated the date when
someone has to leave their own home.

◆ All the ordinary accident-prevention strategies that are
used in everyone's home, including smoke and carbon
monoxide detectors, must be correctly installed, with
working batteries properly fitted or wired into the

electrical system. Stoves and ovens are a particular concern. It is possible to arrange the hob so that the person in the house cannot switch it on randomly and so that it always switches itself off after a short period of use. Devices such as heat alarms have their place, but they may be problematic if the person with dementia does not understand the meaning of the noise when the alarm sounds and fails to exit the house in an emergency.

◆ Medication alerts are among the personal electronic devices that are useful in managing dementia.

I've got two bits of kit I recommend. One is a pillbox. You have to turn it upside down to take the pills out and when you do that an electronic alert signal to your family (for example, your daughter, at work) is cancelled. If you don't knock out the pills at the right time, she gets an alert advising her to phone you about it. The second is a Magiplug. If you put the plug in the sink and turn on the water, and then forget about it, the plug will automatically drain the sink before it overflows. I give that one to students for Christmas. (Dementia nurse)

◆ Technology is not without its problems. It has to be acquired and maintained, and people with dementia have to consent to its being used in their own home. Some of the devices are possibly irritating or even bewildering. If you have always lived alone, a voice coming from seemingly nowhere asking you about your keys or if you need help might be frightening rather than reassuring, particularly if you have forgotten about installing that piece of equipment.

Some electronic inventions are dazzling, but they can only be one part of the answer to the challenge of maintaining the dignity and autonomy of the person with dementia. Body-worn fall detectors are important, but if they are left dangling on the bedpost they don't help when the person falls on the stairs.

What to do in the bedroom

◆ Sleep is really important in dementia. The condition is crushingly tiring and so the person with dementia needs to rest. If they don't sleep at night it causes health and well-being problems for the people who live with them which are so serious that it can precipitate the person having to be admitted to hospital or a care home. The design of the bedroom can help. And of course you also need to think about all the common strategies, like plenty of exercise and daylight during the day, followed by a bedtime routine that involves winding down and perhaps having a warm drink (see Chapter 7 on sleeplessness).

◆ Bedrooms are for relaxing, sleeping and doing intimate things. It's best to keep entertaining and communication equipment such as televisions and computers elsewhere. Remember the evidence that the light from screens falling on the retina of your eyes affects the body clock negatively.

◆ People sleep best where it is dark and quiet and where the room is slightly cooler and the bed warm. From a practical point of view, how you achieve this depends on the design of your house and the time of year. Blackout curtains and blinds can help in summer.

◆ Put away daytime objects such as clothes to reduce the possibility of the person getting up and getting dressed for the day prematurely.

◆ The commonest reason for getting out of bed is to use the toilet. A commode (a moveable item of furniture that has a pot in it, to be used like a toilet) is handy for people with restricted mobility, but when you've got dementia you might not recognise it for what it is, as it is an unfamiliar object that you'd have to learn to use.

◆ It is not usual to label drawers or put up signs, but it might just be that these things will help the person find what they want when they get up in the night.

◆ Get a full night's sleep yourself as a caregiver by using electronic equipment to monitor the person. You can relax, confident that if anything untoward happens you will soon know about it. Sleep deprivation in caregivers may have detrimental effects on your immune system, whether you have reduced quality or duration of sleep. Some people sleep better in bed beside their husband or wife with dementia. Others can only get a decent sleep if they move into another room. The emotional significance of such a move is not to be underestimated.

I bought my mum a baby alarm. It's the same model we use for our small children. She had been sleeping on the sofa downstairs beside Dad in case he needed her in the night. Now she can go up to bed and get a decent sleep. They both look better already. (Danielle, daughter)

Bathrooms and toilets

◆ Incontinence can be a problem in dementia, but it is not inevitable in everyone. In the early stages it is most likely to be caused by not being able to get to the toilet in time. The person might forget to go, or they might not leave enough time to get there and get out of their clothes. It's potentially embarrassing and inconvenient. In some cases it is caused by, or made worse because of, difficulty in finding and using the toilet. There is further discussion about various aspects of finding the toilet throughout the book.

◆ If your house is a perfect design there will be an en-suite toilet in the bedroom in addition to a downstairs toilet for convenience if the bedroom is upstairs. The en suite toilet will have the toilet pan positioned where it can be seen from the head of the bed, and you'll have a movement sensor that switches on the light when you get out of bed. The toilet seat colour will contrast with the floor and walls and the rest of the bathroom furniture. That's the ideal, so that is what you should expect in a newly designed care home or specifically designed housing, but there are ways round less perfect conditions in your own home. There is a balance to be struck between having enough light to find the toilet and it being dark enough to promote good sleep. It depends on what the person is used to.

One inventor came to me with a prototype 'glow in the dark' luminous toilet seat. I didn't really think it was a great idea for dementia; it was too unfamiliar. (Dementia nurse)

◆ Mirrors can cause problems – particularly in the bathroom, where they are required for grooming – if the person does not recognise their face any more.

◆ Light should be bright, but avoid glare. Contrasting colours in grab bars, toilet seats, hand towels, and so on are really helpful for people to see. Shiny floors should be avoided as they appear to be wet and can make the area seem dangerous. Watch out for other reflective and shiny surfaces, which can cause problems with glare or reflections that are not understood. It is not only mirrors that cause problems.

◆ Wash-hand basins and baths should have classic designs of taps (faucets) so that they are easy to recognise and to use.

In our local Harvey Nicks there is a gorgeous ladies' toilet but my problem is the fancy taps. I twist them this way and that, often with soapy hands, and I can't work out whether you are supposed to use it like a lever or a knob. They're a miracle of Continental fashion and design but I can't work them. (Jane, 59)

◆ Bathtub and sink plugs can be replaced with Magiplugs to avoid flooding accidents. We've seen places where people are not allowed to have a plug for fear of causing an overflow of water on to the floor. This little product has a pressure sensor in it so that if the water gets too deep, it releases the water down the drain. Hot water can cause scalding. Centrally control the maximum temperature for hot water to avoid accidents.

◆ Sort out the lock on the door so that you will be able
to get in if assistance is needed; an outward-opening
door might help with that as well. As we have seen,
contrasting colours for grab bars are important.
Remove items such as toilet-roll holders if you suspect
the person is using them as a grab bar, as they might
come off the wall and cause a fall.

Kitchens and dining rooms

◆ Good design of the kitchen and dining room is
vital for a person with dementia because eating and
drinking are especially important for their health.
In other chapters you will see how failing to eat and
drink properly can lead to health problems, such as
infections, falls and confusion – any of which can result
in an admission to hospital, from which the person
may never return to their own home. It is crucial to
adapt the kitchen to allow people with dementia to
enjoy food as much as possible for as long as possible.

*When I was training to be a nurse we were taught that
dementia was a 'wasting disease' and people got 'cachexia',
which meant they withered away and died. I realised later,
to my horror, that the main problem was that they never got
enough to eat. (Jane, 59)*

◆ Your aim should be that the person is able to continue
to make meals for themselves and visitors for as long
as possible, even if they are quite simple meals. When
a person with dementia goes into hospital, they may
have to undertake a kitchen assessment before being

'allowed' to go home by the health and social care system. It's often undertaken by an occupational therapist. The sooner the dementia-friendly ideas are incorporated in their own kitchen the better. This will allow any of us to become used to our dementia-friendly kitchen before it is too late. The design of the kitchen can help you pass the test.

◆ There are design features that will encourage eating and drinking. These could include having a glass-fronted fridge so that all the tasty things are on view, or glass-fronted cupboards where the bright and attractive packaging of all the nutritious items is visible.

I find the secret is to do the opposite of what the slimming magazines recommend. They suggest keeping fattening foods out of sight. I recommend keeping them in full view – creating temptation. (Ellen, dietician)

◆ You can also use a little plug-in electric machine called an Ode, which will release at carefully timed intervals selected food odours that have been shown to make people hungry and more interested in eating. Combine this with the glass-door fridge that allows the person with dementia to see tasty treats and helps tempt them to eat. The glass door also makes it easier for a family member or care worker to check if food is going off and needs clearing out. You might find such fridges marketed as wine coolers in stores or online retailers – just get different shelves.

◆ Keeping people involved with cooking is a good way of encouraging them to eat. You have to be sure that health and safety and food hygiene concerns don't take precedence over normal living. Careful planning helps, and looking out for the available assistive technology, such as microwaves with barcode readers so you don't have to read the print on the packaging, which is always too small. Another useful device is the induction hob that remains cool to the touch while heating up cooking pots. Most of these induction units have safety functions that will shut them off if the pan is empty or there is no appropriate pot on the stove.

◆ When designing the kitchen, you need to consider all the issues outlined elsewhere in this book about flooring and lighting. As ever, keeping the lighting bright is important. Trip hazards need to be considered and floor colours and coverings that support safe walking are needed. There are commercially available floor coverings that are easy to clean and will retain a high level of slip resistance even when wet and others that are frankly risky. Carpet may be hard to clean in the kitchen but it does have the advantage of being softer in the case of falls. Cleanable carpets and replaceable carpet tiles offer practical solutions. Remember that the culprit in the fall is often the footwear as much as the floor.

◆ Total risk-avoidance is seriously limiting, but often kitchen risks can be reduced by the use of technology. There needs to be a serious discussion about what level of risk is acceptable and to whom, as the estimation of the risk seems to vary hugely between hospital-based and community-based professional staff, with hospital staff having a bias against the person's own home. There are devices on the market that may reassure anxious relatives and neighbours who are afraid of accidents and falls. It is important to emphasise the right of the person with dementia to choose to take risks and not be deprived of their liberty. When the point is reached where the stove cannot be used safely, disconnect it, or remove the knobs if knob covers are not available. This is preferable to moving the person out of their home.

◆ Declutter the kitchen and put away things that are not often used, leaving out the stuff that is most likely to be used regularly, such as the kettle, tea bags and cookie jar. Keeping things handy will discourage people from climbing on the furniture to reach high cupboards. Consider taking the doors off the front of some cupboard units or fitting glass doors so that contents can be found without too much searching. Anything that is out of the way is less likely to be used (appropriately or inappropriately). Remember the declutter/forgetting problem and be prepared to handle questions or confusion about where possessions have gone. Anything that is poisonous and could cause harm could be removed altogether.

◆ When appliances need to be replaced, buy the same brand and model if possible to help the person to continue to be able to use it. Keep the electric kettle away from the stove to reduce the chance of the person putting it on there by mistake. The first time that happens, get rid of it and buy a stovetop kettle. A whistle is needed if the kettle does not automatically shut off.

Living areas

◆ Internal spaces like living rooms, hallways and stairs present challenges. People with dementia will be moving round the house with a variety of purposes, sometimes at night when they are tired and sleepy. Sometimes there will be a sense of urgency, as when they are going to the bathroom. Worn or loose carpets have to be sorted and banisters are best if they are on both sides of the stairs. People make mistakes about where the edges of furniture are, so sharp corners on furniture could be sanded down. Low coffee tables can be dangerous.

◆ The light switches should contrast markedly with the wall to make finding them easier. If the person has lived in the house for a long time, they may reach for the light switch without even looking, so this advice is even more important for custom-built supportive housing. You can make a significant improvement in visibility by changing the base plate of the switch or by framing it on the wall with some brightly coloured tape or other contrasting decorative material.

◆ The general principles about contrasting furniture and contrasts between walls and flooring that are described in other sections also apply here.

Outdoors

They offered us a place in a day centre, but what Dad really wanted was a buddy to take him up to the allotment and back; who would keep quiet and leave him in peace while he was there. (Daughter of J., 82)

◆ Going outside is really important for people with dementia. Chapter 6 explains how important exercise and exposure to daylight are for mood and sleep. There is a clear connection between vitamin D deficiency and falls, and the best source of vitamin D is sunlight on skin. Setting the body clock is only one of the benefits of getting outside.

◆ Pottering in the garden is a great way to stay well. Even if you don't have a garden you can get a great deal of pleasure from a balcony with pot plants on it, and a chair on which to sit and look out. A balcony is not automatically dangerous for a person with dementia, depending on what they are used to and the design of the balcony.

◆ If the family is concerned about the person with dementia leaving the garden and getting lost, it is possible to reduce the risk by having the right sort of fence or boundary. The gate in the fence can be made unobtrusive with planting or by putting the fastenings on the outside. It is also possible to put a fence halfway across the garden so that the person does have a gate that they can go in and out of at will.

◆ The garden or yard is a great way of distracting people who may be agitated or distressed, because there is always something to do, whether it is weeding, sweeping paths, digging, grass cutting or even hanging out the washing. It offers additional benefits because the skills used outside have been there for a long time. There is great satisfaction to be had in showing young people how to do something like potting up a plant or taking a cutting.

To forget how to dig the earth and to tend the soil is to forget ourselves. (Mahatma Gandhi)

chapter 10

Eating, drinking and dementia

The more fit and well you feel, whether you are a person with dementia or a caregiver, the better you will be able to handle the unexpected situations and stresses that arise which could, if handled badly, lead to the person with dementia going downhill. There is more advice in Chapter 3 for caregivers on how to stay well.

Eating and drinking properly can make a lot of difference. Keeping a healthy diet going can be challenging at the best of times, but it is really important to maintain the strength and health of everyone in the house by making sure of regular meals. If this is difficult, you could consider a meal delivery service. There are private companies that will deliver meals direct. You might go out more for meals, because that is not necessarily overly expensive.

We go to the supermarket café every day for lunch. We don't need a lot so we have the 'kid's meal' (they laugh when they give me the coloring book, but I save them up for the grandchildren). It's good to have a cooked meal once a day and I don't have to do all the preparation and wash up. It gets us out, and I see a lot of the same people there each day. The ladies at the till are getting to know us. It is much cheaper than the meals on wheels because we can choose what we fancy each day and nothing gets wasted or thrown away. (D., 83)

Many women of an older generation relied on their husbands for driving and if he is the person with dementia the transport problems can be considerable. For food shopping, consider using the online shopping and delivery service from a supermarket. If you are not confident with that, you may have someone in the family who will help you and in some areas the local authority or a voluntary organisation provides a low-cost shopping service.

I know one lady in the North of England with a daughter in Canada who does her weekly shop for the mom online, and it gets delivered as regular as clockwork. That's very good, but we have set up a local social enterprise and we do it using volunteers for people who don't have families. (community worker)

While on the subject of eating and drinking, staying hydrated is really important. It is not unusual for older people to selectively avoid drinking in order to try to reduce the need to use the toilet. This is not clever. You need water for all your bodily functions, including your blood supply, and if you allow yourself to get dry you will lose some of your cognitive functions. If you've already got some dementia symptoms, dehydration will make the situation worse. You will get confused. It is also very likely that you will develop a urinary tract infection (sometimes called a UTI) and get even more confused as a result. You can end up in hospital just from not drinking enough water, and this is particularly true if you are already coming down with dementia. Keep your pee a nice pale straw colour. If it gets any darker drink more. If it gets smelly see a doctor as fast as you can to get antibiotics before you end up in an ambulance. Water is the stuff of life. So drink some. Tea is also good. In fact almost any fluid helps, and you get fluid from other food, like soups and custard.

Complications around eating and drinking

At times it can be more difficult to get someone with dementia to take the right amount of the right food. This section is about the practical issues involved with getting them to eat, even if they don't seem to have much appetite for food.

Eating and drinking are essential for life, and a source of great pleasure for most of us. As outlined before, a person with dementia might begin to have difficulty with shopping and cooking food by themselves, and when that happens their diet can suffer. But as time goes by their dementia might mean they find it difficult to recognise and enjoy food, and so they will require help to make sure they have a good diet. Practical things can be done to make it more likely that people with dementia will continue to enjoy their food for as long as possible and get the benefit of a good diet and fluids.

There is a current fad for a weight-loss diet that involves eating only a small amount of calories over twenty-four hours twice a week. Even if you take a normal diet on the other five days you will lose weight. If a person with dementia misses eating properly on only two days in the week, it is as if they are on this diet. It is no surprise that under these circumstances the person will lose weight at a time in life when that is not desirable for most people.

Drinking

In any emergency lack of fluid is always more serious than lack of food. A young, healthy and fit person can survive without fluid for a few days, and without food for a few weeks, but they'll not be very well.

Not having enough to drink can cause deterioration in a person with dementia much more quickly. The brain ceases to work well in anyone who is dehydrated at any age. In the past, children in school were never offered fluids during classes, but it is now recognised that they learn better if they have easy access to drinking water. For someone with dementia who is already struggling with their thinking, not having enough to drink can quickly make them more confused.

How much is needed depends on the person's metabolism and their activity, and the temperature in which they are living, set by the heating in their home or the weather outside. You can tell if the person has not had enough to drink usually from their urine becoming dark and concentrated, and from their skin losing its flexibility. People can die of dehydration very fast, like someone who exercises in the sun, or a baby locked in a hot car. A person with dementia who is dehydrating over a matter of days will have sunken eyes and a dry mouth. The heartbeat becomes more rapid and the person lethargic. It's very serious.

The person is more likely to drink if there are lots of cues. Have the kettle and teapot in full view along with the tea bags. If you have a glass-door fridge, have lots of attractive bottles of juice on show. Keep jugs of water and glasses somewhere convenient. Suggest a drink at every opportunity. Have drinks on the table at mealtimes. Just reminding the person to drink has great value. Suggest having a drink every time you talk to the person with dementia.

Junior doctors in hospitals should carry a glass of water and offer a sip to the patient in between questions when interviewing them. The nurses are so busy and the person has so little support to stay hydrated. It is the least they can do. (Hospital consultant)

Dehydration in hospital is very common for practical reasons. If the person staying at home is allowed to get dehydrated, the danger is that they will end up in a hospital that only makes the situation worse for them.

What should people drink? In general anything is better than nothing, but of course water is very good. For younger people water is best, but for older people in particular, if their appetite is poor, you have to be sure that you are not filling them up with so much water that they can't eat enough. Make sure in those cases that they are drinking things that offer calories and vitamins – for example, a milkshake or fresh fruit juice. Tea and coffee with caffeine in them might be limited towards the end of the day if you want to reduce nocturnal wandering, but they are great first thing in the morning when people wake up. If the person has blood pressure problems, then they may have to have decaffeinated drinks. The amount of fluid needed depends on what you are doing and how hot the environment is. Hospitals can get very hot, even if you are sitting still all the time. Alcohol can be nice, but you need to be sure that it is not interfering with medication, so get approval first from the doctor and remember that the smaller and older you are, the less you can tolerate alcohol. Used in excess it also causes dehydration.

Going to the bathroom can be complicated at times, and it has been said already that it is not unusual for people with dementia to deliberately reduce their fluid intake to avoid the complication of having to get to the toilet in a hurry. The problem with this is that it will lead to some increase in their dementia symptoms, and if they do it long enough they will get a urinary tract infection (UTI), or a 'chill on the bladder', that will cause even more confusion and can lead to a hospital admission for intravenous antibiotics, as we have already seen. It is a shame to end up on a 'drip' or IV line because you were trying to avoid wetting yourself. If continence is an issue, people need to be directed to the continence nurse who you can find via the doctor to get assessment and support, and discreet pads if needed. Danger of incontinence should not be a problem that leads to people avoiding fluids.

Take particular care when the person with dementia goes into hospital or a care home.

When my mom was in hospital they put her water jug where she could not reach it. She could not even see it, of course, because it was clear, and the water was clear and so was the beaker. I put it within her reach and put a bit of orange cordial in it, and she helped herself after that. (Jane, daughter of D., 85)

Eating

We were always taught that dementia was a wasting disease ... people lost weight rapidly in the old psychiatric hospital before they died. (Dementia nurse)

It was not necessary in most cases for those people to lose weight. Of course, towards the very end of life, as the body closes down and the person is dying, there is a natural process that takes place, but people with dementia in the past were quite simply not fed properly in institutions. Learning from what went wrong then can give us a clue about how to do it properly at home. The power you have when the person is in their own home means that you can avoid these hazards.

The problems encountered in care homes included:

◆ rigid mealtimes that came and went whether you were hungry or not;

◆ no choice over what was served or influence over the menu;

◆ food served in uncomfortable surroundings and in unattractive servings;

◆ too much or too little served on the plate;

◆ more than one course stacked on the tray or table at the same time;

◆ nothing to eat between meals;

◆ a long fast from 'tea' or 'supper' at 5.30 p.m. until breakfast at 8 a.m.;

◆ no allowances made for the changes in dementia;

◆ no allowances made for sensory and physical impairments;

◆ hurried shovelling of food into people who needed help to eat;

◆ use of sedation, so people were too drowsy to eat;

◆ uneaten food removed without keeping a record, or weighing the person regularly.

We could not work out why Florence would not eat in the care home. When I sat with her she eventually whispered, 'I've got no money ... I'm not able to pay for this.' She thought she was in a restaurant or hotel and because they had taken away her handbag she thought she was going to be embarrassed by a bill. At every mealtime we got into the habit of discreetly letting her know that it was all paid for in advance and she could take as much as she wanted. (Care worker)

Mealtimes

The person with dementia may not wish to eat when it is 'time to eat'. Some prefer to graze throughout the day, never actually wanting to sit down at a table.

I keep a cookie jar and bowls of sweets around the

place all the time, as well as bananas and nice soft fruit like strawberries. I see Mum just going up and helping herself. I've got a fridge with wrapped tiny sandwiches and savouries that I can produce at a moment's notice if she fancies one. (Daughter of 76-year-old woman with dementia)

Food should be available at any time, night or day. You can make this possible in your own home in simple practical ways. Of course there are limitations to when food may be available in hospitals and care homes, and the tyranny of food hygiene control has at times meant that people have been starving in those settings because the risk of food poisoning was overestimated.

We used to give them scrambled eggs in the evening if they were peckish, but now we are not allowed because of fear of salmonella. (Nurse)

If the person eats well at home, you need to investigate whether you can supply them with food for snacking if you have to temporarily leave them in a hospital or care home.

If for important reasons you would like the person at home to eat at a particular time – for example, because that is the only time you are available to support them by cooking or assisting them to eat – there are practical things that can help:

◆ Cue the fact that it is time to eat by creating smells of cooking artificially or naturally. Machines that emit appetite-stimulating smells are available commercially, or perhaps this can happen in the ordinary way through cooking and maybe involving the person with dementia in the cooking. Preparing a meal can make you hungry. Fried-onion smells will make people buy hot dogs that taste of virtually nothing, so why not use cooking onions as an appetite stimulant for your nourishing meals? The smell of vanilla or of baking bread is famously mouthwatering. The smell of toasting fruit bread is said to be particularly appetizing.

◆ If eating at a table is what the person prefers, set the table formally and make it attractive, using napkins and cruets, then get them to sit up at the table on a comfortable chair. Other people prefer a tray on their lap – everyone is different and you need to do what works.

◆ Use contrasting crockery so that the food can be seen on the plate and stands out from the tabletop, tray or tablecloth. A portion of white potatoes with white fish, on a white plate with a white tablecloth, may be almost invisible to a person with depth-perception problems and ageing eyes.

◆ Reduce distractions by switching off the radio and television, and focusing on the food. Make sure there is lots of light on the food.

◆ Eat with the person with dementia. Eating is a social activity.

Mealtimes that are pleasant help with good digestion. Taking time is also important.

Dr Kevin Charras in research in a care home introduced a

very long lunchtime where everyone took about an hour and a half to eat a number of courses. Everyone put on weight. What was the point of rushing? There was little else to do. (Report from J.M. on research from Fondation Médéric Alzheimer)

Choice

The simplest ideas are often the best. If you want someone to eat, offer them what they really, really like.

For days on end Dad only seemed to want to eat custard and bananas. Not a very balanced diet and an odd thing to ask for first thing in the morning. He was not interested in eggs or cheese, or steak pies or all his usual favourite things. The community psychiatric nurse reassured me that I should just give him what he wanted in the meantime and only worry if it went on for weeks. In the end he started to refuse the custard and was asking for other things, and no harm seemed to come of it. I just felt a bit guilty. (Daughter of 70-year-old man)

It is important to stay calm and flexible about eating and drinking. If you are a member of the family or a friend you probably know what the person prefers to eat and drink, and when.

Common problems of ageing and stress

A general reduction in the sense of taste and smell in old people can become greater with dementia. People sometimes find it hard to have a family meal and eat alongside people with later stages of dementia if they are displaying behavioural problems at mealtimes, including playing with food, refusing to eat it or spitting it out. There may be several reasons for this.

I got to know with Mom that if she did not like something she'd just spit it back at me. I learned not to try new flavors or textures. Eventually it was as if she had forgotten how to eat, or chew or swallow. (Sarah, daughter of Alice, 92)

In other cases the person may become agitated and angry at mealtimes because of a combination of difficulties.

Gordon hated eating with other people. He felt as if he was being watched by them, and he hated the loss of dignity because we had to help him spoon his food to his mouth. With the Lewy body dementia he got a bit paranoid and at times he actually thought the food might be poisoned. (Alison, wife of Gordon, 68)

Trying to make mealtimes as enjoyable and stress-free as possible is an art. One important element is the place, and the accessibility of the table and chair. People who are eating in groups may feel under stress to complete their food at the same time as others, even if they are still a little bit hungry, so watch for that when eating out. Cutlery is available with different larger handles, for ease of use, and there are cups and mugs specifically designed to cope with practical problems in older people, such as the weight of the cup, the size and balance of the handle, and whether it is easy to grasp in two hands. Non-slip placemats can help prevent plates from moving around, and a plate with a lip on the edge can help prevent food from sliding off the plate altogether. But don't go overboard.

I hated seeing my mother being offered food on plastic plates. We've found some attractive colored pottery that meets her needs and we don't mind if it gets broken. Plastic is for babies and for picnics, not a hot dinner for a lady of eighty. (Sarah, daughter of Alice, 92)

Dementia changes

In some cases, enjoyment of food decreases as the dementia increases. The person may seem to lose interest in eating and drinking. It is not just that they 'forget' to eat and drink. Their appetite might seem to be poor even if food is put in front of them. It is important to be aware of the sorts of problems that might arise and have some practical ideas about possible solutions. People get quite upset if they have prepared a meal and it is rejected. There is a lot of emotion attached to food.

If as a result of the dementia the person is taking less exercise, this can give rise to constipation, which will in turn reduce appetite. Make sure that plenty of fluids are taken and ensure that the diet includes fibre. The loss of appetite and constipation can be made worse by painkillers or the side effects of other medicines. Check with the doctor, nurse or pharmacist. When the person has dementia they might not tell you that they are in pain. For example, a poorly fitting denture or a sore mouth might not get mentioned to you, but the person just stops eating.

It is quite common for people with dementia to have depression in addition. Depression can reduce appetite. It is important to get it diagnosed and treated. Try to keep the person involved in choosing and preparing food to keep up interest and check that you are giving them 'a little of what they fancy'.

Familiarity and routine are important for a person with dementia, and so when planning meals you should take this into consideration. Some people with dementia pace around and use up a lot of energy, and in those cases you may want to enrich their diet in order to get enough calories into them. One way of doing this is to add calories to what they would normally eat and drink. If your dad normally eats porridge made with salt and water, add some cream to the recipe.

If the person you are trying to support is older and frail, they may have a smaller appetite and eat sparingly, which means you have to get all the calories and vitamins they need into smaller amounts of food. Nearly everyone knows the difference between fattening and non-fattening foods these days. For a person who does not eat much, the richer the food the better. They still need the fibre that comes from vegetables, but you can dress them with rich sauces, or butter, to keep the calories high.

When we have mashed potatoes I make them with cream and butter. My mother eats like a bird, but I can tempt her with little pots of full-fat yoghurt and as many chocolate gingers as she wants. (Daughter living at home with her mother)

Difficulty in swallowing can affect people with dementia. This can be associated with a loss of coordination skills. It might help if you think about the mechanics of chewing and swallowing. First the food has to get into your mouth, poor eyesight or difficulties with cutlery can be a problem in achieving that. Then you have to manipulate it into a soft ball of food that can be swallowed, and this requires saliva, which may be reduced in old age and with some medicines or dehydration. Sore gums and mouth ulcers or poor teeth can be a problem, so you need to get the dentist to take a look. The tongue then coordinates pushing the food back into the throat without allowing it to go into the lungs, which could cause choking. A speech therapist can advise on what sort of consistency of food is best at various stages of dementia. To begin with, keep going with everything that is popular. In the end, perhaps some items need to be softened. Curiously, mixed textures in one mouthful are sometimes a problem, like soup with bits, or crunchy cereal in milk.

The perfect meal

A great meal is when everyone is relaxed and happy, with the food that is served to your taste and in exactly the right amounts. You've got enough time to eat it and, if you have company, enough time to socialise over it, and you are not worrying about how it is going to be paid for. The surroundings are comfortable and you are not distracted by noise or harassed by the people serving the meal. Any faux pas like dropping your cutlery, or having to spit out an unexpected bone or olive stone, can be overcome discreetly, and any spills or drips are dealt with using your lovely big napkin. Many care homes achieve this with people who are very disabled by their dementia, but some do not, and hospitals are notoriously unfocused on this issue. You may need to keep an eye on this for your loved one even while they are at home. And if the person can't sit still for a whole meal, finger food and snacking are great ways to get enough calories in, washed down by frequent hot and cold drinks, available on demand. Bon appetit!

chapter 11

What to look for in residential care

Care in a care home

It used to be that care homes were retirement homes for relatively active people who could not or would not care for themselves. In general now between 70 and 90 per cent of care home residents have dementia, and the average length of stay in most parts of the UK has dropped to eighteen months. So the care home is more often like a hospice for people with dementia and very frail people at the end of their life.

The form of early-onset dementia that Alan had is quite unusual. We live in a rural area and there was not a specialist unit nearby. Complex and unusual cases had to travel a long way to a centre that covered a wide geographical area. Apparently families often have to rely on local services targeted at older people, even if the person with dementia is younger. (Widow of Alan, 55)

Some people never have to go into a residential facility. But if you do, what is available and what this is called varies around the world. Here is the definition from the Alzheimer's Association of the USA:

Nursing homes (also called skilled nursing facility, long-term care facility, custodial care):

Nursing homes provide round-the-clock care and long-term medical treatment. Most nursing homes have services and staff to address issues such as nutrition, care planning, recreation, spirituality and medical care. Different nursing homes have different staff-to-resident ratios. Also, the staff at one nursing home may have more experience or training with dementia than the staff at another. Nursing homes are usually licensed by the state and regulated by the federal government. (Alzheimer's Association, USA)

The names that are given to residential facilities reflect a different cultural approach in each country. In many countries the term 'custodial care' is used only for the secure unit that might house a person with a criminal conviction. The laws on the use of restraint and the protection of vulnerable adults are quite clear about when it is, and is not, permissible to lock someone up, even if it is what the family would wish for, but the observance of those rules is not always well monitored. In some places there are differences between care homes and nursing homes and dementia specialist homes but in general they all provide for people with dementia at earlier or later stages.

In Australia, facilities are described as providing high level, low level and dementia-specific care. People with dementia might reside in any of these three government funded units, but many people in high level care are in the later stages of dementia. The dementia-specific unit has the capacity to care for people safely when they have significant additional needs. Deciding where you stay depends on an assessment called an ACAT (Aged Care Assessment Team). The doctor or hospital can help you to contact the local ACAT, or you can find it on the Agedcare Australia website (http://www.myagedcare.gov.au/)

Alzheimer's Australia says:

The ACAT will determine the level of care needed by the person with dementia. The team will assess their needs and recommend appropriate types of residential care and provide details of facilities which may be suitable. Any concerns or issues that you may have can be discussed with the team. As applications will usually have to be made to several facilities it may be necessary to visit many places. Try to work through the list of facilities in an organised way taking notes as you go. If possible, take a friend or family member on the visits. Trust your intuition and common sense when assessing residential care facilities for a person with dementia. (Alzheimer's Australia)

Choosing a care home is one of the most expensive and emotional decisions you will ever have to make, and it is hard to know what is best and how to work out if the home is continuing to provide what is needed afterwards. In this chapter we'll go into what a good care home looks like and the financial considerations. If you were to believe all the frightening news stories that abound, you'd naturally be pessimistic about the possibility of having a good time in a care home, or being content to let your parent or spouse go to live in one.

Far too many care homes are dumps, in every sense of the word … Last year six 'carers' at the Winterbourne View home in Bristol were jailed for 'cruel, callous and degrading' abuse of elderly residents. This awful place is unlikely to be unique. Why are we afraid of ending our lives in care? Because far too many care homes are … uncaring, shabby places that are incapable of showing human compassion when it is needed the most. (Tony Parsons, from 'Why I'd rather die in Dignitas than live in the torture chambers of a British care home', Mirror, 2 March 2013)

The number of people who end up in a care home is relatively small, but it varies for reasons that are not related to a measure of dependency. For example, across the four countries of the UK which are very similar in respect – Scotland, England, Northern Ireland and Wales – there is great variation. It is not only the availability of community services or the level of dementia that is the primary reason for going to a care home. In general you have less than a 20 per cent chance of ending up in a care home, even if you are over seventy-five. In Northern Ireland, the number of people in care homes in the first decade of the twenty-first century was higher than anywhere else in the UK. The reason for this is not known, but it is probably that families had a positive view of care homes – more positive than Tony Parsons in any case. Also, there may have been less pressure on public spending, meaning that local authorities had budgets that would allow them to make placements at levels unheard of in England. But even in Northern Ireland the government is making huge changes, shutting government operated care homes and increasing the pressure towards care in the community.

You can compare this with Canada. There, 'nursing homes' serve people who don't need to be in hospital, but who do need 24-hour nursing care that would not usually be available in a retirement home. In 2013 there were nearly 1,400 of these in Canada, providing homes for around 200,000 people. Nearly three quarters of the residents were funded by provincial and municipal plans and agencies, but the rest had insurance or paid for themselves with private funds. More than 70 per cent of the homes were private, either for-profit, or non-profit.

Care homes are often the place of last resort when attempts to keep a person at home have failed, and the person has a great need of support towards the end of life. Residents are more often women, partly because women have up till now lived longer and also because, in general, older women at present are more likely to be able to care for their partner or spouse than older men when things go wrong. Make sure your sons are domesticated, because in future they will need to be! Length of stay is declining, and this could be seen as a result of improved community care, increasing cost of care home care acting as a brake, or an increase in older people getting what they want, which is usually to stay at home.

What does good look like?

In many countries there are reporting mechanisms for the standards in care homes. Just as important is how the home seems to you. Phone, write to or email a number of homes and ask about the level of care provided for dementia, the fees (if any) and the waiting lists. You will be able to see recent inspection reports on the inspectors' website or ask the home to send you a copy. Visit the places that are interesting. Websites always look nice. That's what the design company is paid for.

In a good home you will experience friendly greetings, a homely and welcoming atmosphere, a clean and pleasantly decorated environment and the right smell. You will probably have a sense of what is good when you see it, as long as you are not taken in by hotel-type décor that looks elegant but is not suitable for dementia. The first visit is probably best done on your own or with a friend who knows about or has experience of care homes. If you think that the place is promising, you can follow up with the potential resident and see what their reaction is. Some places offer day care or respite, and that would give you a chance to test and try before you make a decision. Some people think about having a trial residential period before signing a contract. It's not clear what the benefit would be. If it is not good, you are going to move the person even if the initial trial was positive. The home is on trial for the whole period that they are caring for your loved one.

The sort of things you are looking for include:

◆ Is everyone treated with dignity and respect? This starts with how you are treated, but when you are visiting, how do staff members refer to residents? Do they talk about 'them' as if 'they' are not there, or do they address residents as respected clients? Do they call them by their name or some general endearment? Are people treated like adults? You would expect to see a written philosophy statement about this and some evidence that it is used in staff training with visible results.

My uncle was Professor John Edmund Baird. Nearly everyone called him Professor Baird. Only his wife and mother had called him anything else and that was 'Edmund'. I discovered the staff were addressing him as 'John' and 'darling' and I was concerned. In a lucid moment he told me, 'I don't want you to tell them my name is Edmund. This way I know who they are – impudent strangers.' (Anne B., niece)

◆ In the public areas, if there is a TV on is anyone watching it, and is the programme relevant to the residents? What are people doing in the day room, and is there a staff member with them? It's not really homely if all the chairs are in a big circle rather than conversation groups. Are residents involved in activities, nicely dressed and groomed, alert and interested? Do residents talk to you? If not they are clearly used to being ignored. Can you see people doing things for themselves – laying tables, reading a book? Of course there may be a tired person sleeping in a chair – but not everyone.

◆ Do the staff and the systems focus on the abilities of the person with dementia? It is probably quicker and easier to dress and feed someone than to help them to do it for themselves. If a staff member makes the decision for them about this, is it in the interest of the resident with dementia? You need to ask them some questions about dementia and judge their answers for yourself. Not least, ask them what training they've had.

◆ Everyone should have a care plan that is regularly reviewed; staff should all have recognised training in care planning. A large part of that is the importance of meaningful activity. The care plan should include as much as possible of the person's life story so that their routines and relationships can be respected and maintained. Does the plan single out one worker who is the key contact for the resident, taking a particular interest and looking out for them consistently over time?

◆ Do staff knock and wait for more than a heartbeat for a reply before entering rooms? Dignity and privacy are not preserved if the knocking and entering are all in one swift movement. It is a good clue when staff are showing you round if they take you into a resident's room, even in their absence, without asking permission. Watch how staff talk to each other and to residents while you are there. Remember, this is when the care home providers are on their best behaviour.

◆ Will the resident be able to choose their food, and when they eat? What happens if they are hungry or fancy a hot drink in between mealtimes? Can you share a meal with them, or make some tea?

They showed me a sample lunch menu and I asked if there was a vegetarian option. The cook replied, 'Oh, we have that at supper time.' (J.A., home visitor)

◆ What opportunities are there for exercise and outdoor activities? Is the garden open access and with a dementia-friendly design, including things to do and see, places to sit, and safe walking. Are there any animals, like chickens or rabbits? You'd expect there to be an active programme of external visits, whether that is visiting a café or pub, or going somewhere interesting, like a local park or the seaside. And how is it recorded? You're not interested in how many times there is a trip to the seaside. You want to know how many times your relative will be on one.

I asked if there were any parties or events, and they described a Royal Baby party in great detail. When I asked if Esme took part they said it was a shame because she was not well that day. It almost felt deceitful and it certainly would have been misleading if I had not asked the second question. (Legal representative and attorney)

◆ In the bedroom is there space for personal possessions and for storage? You need a place for at least two people to sit and chat. An interesting view can be really important. I know that people are anxious about balconies, but at the Dementia Services Development Centre (www.dementia.stir.ac.uk) we like them, if they are properly designed and used.

◆ What is done about security? If there is a resident who tends to abscond, it is wrong to lock everyone else up. Use of assistive technology by the home is to be expected for this purpose. Are they so obsessed with security that you can't open a window and get fresh air? Air quality is really important. No one wants to live out their days in a stuffy atmosphere.

◆ Does the home respect cultural differences of clients in both activities and behaviour of staff? Can people maintain relationships with the outside world and the community within which they were living before the care home?

◆ End of life care is a very important issue. It is never too soon to talk about what is to happen.

I was a bit shocked when Dad was moving in and they asked me what was to happen when he died. I mean, of course he was going to die, but they were asking all about funeral directors, cremation etc. If he got ill and there was not much hope did I want him moved to a hospital, or what? When the time came and he did die I was so glad we had got all that over with. They were so comforting and helpful and it really made a very difficult experience easier for me and my mother. (H.B., son)

The building

The Dementia Services Development Centre at the University of Stirling has discovered an interesting anomaly in the design of care home buildings. Over twenty-five years of supporting dementia-friendly design, we have found that what appeals to those who are choosing a care home is not necessarily the same as what works well for people with dementia. A home designed to look like a country house hotel, with soft lighting, subtle colour schemes, gilded mirrors, and hidden and discreet toilet facilities, leading off to corridors with rows of identical hotel room doors, will win industry prizes. However much this style appeals to families and people making decisions on behalf of others, it may not be right for people with dementia, according to the research.

To help a person with dementia the ideal design is much brighter and more obvious. A big coloured toilet door just off the dining room helps avoid the problem of being 'caught short' during a meal. The effect of light on the person's capacity to work out what is going on has already been emphasised, so bright light is needed. You don't want elegant drapes and pelmets across the windows if they reduce daylight. Highly contrasting floor coverings and wall coverings are important to help with mobility and visual impairments, including problems with depth perception. This might not seem so comfortable or even luxurious at first. It's more kids' show Balamory than Queen Elizabeth's Balmoral. Balamory is a kids' show on TV and Balmoral is Queen Elizabeth's Scottish castle. More nursery school than country house. But it is more useful than elegant, and given the choice, people with dementia need all the useful help they can get.

In discussion it is often said that not everyone in a care home has dementia and so homes don't all need this. The sad truth is that with the reduction in public resources for care and the increasing cost of care, no one is funded to go into a care home until they are quite frail. Research is starting to show that around 90 per cent of care home residents in Scotland have dementia even in care homes that do not claim to specialise in this form of care. Where people once lived in care homes for years, as we've seen, a residential lifetime of eighteen months is now more likely, and many residents do not reach that milestone. The chances are that in future the care home resident in general will be frail, very elderly and have at the very least the early stages of dementia.

The dementia-friendly design concept is based on a mixture of research involving people with dementia, extrapolation from the needs of people with sensory and physical impairment, and knowledge of what the international consensus is on best practice. The dementia-friendly building is comfortable and elegant, but not in the way that people might think if they have a Victorian stately home in mind. The person is unlikely only to have dementia and may also have other illnesses and impairments that come with great age.

There are care homes which are focused on the needs of a particular social group or cultural community, such as military veterans' homes, or care homes for Jewish or Polish people. They should have design features that reflect the history and culture of the residents in general. However, because the home is only ever going to be 'home' to any individual for a short time, it has to follow certain general rules, while offering the maximum flexibility in the resident's own space. If the home has to be homogeneous and work for a lot of different people, let it at least be based on research evidence about what works, and not this season's palette from the interior design fashion magazines.

Being 'dementia friendly' is not the same as winning a prize for design, because architecture and design prizes are given for a range of reasons that may not be related to dementia design principles. If you want to compare the home you are seeing with a high dementia-specific standard, there are examples of ideal dementia environments at https://www2.health.vic.gov.au/ageing-and-aged-care/dementia-friendly-environments. This resource was produced by the Victoria State Government in Australia for use in residential care facilities, but the information and advice is useful for any space.

Homes should offer a domestic-like environment. This means that if it is quite large, it should be divided down into smaller units. Ensuite facilities are required in many places for all new and newly registered care buildings. People should share a room only by choice and no more than two people at a time. If two are sharing they should have another room for their personal use – as it were, a bedroom and a living room. All the design features highlighted in Chapter 9 work for care home settings. The judicious use of assistive technology means that even if you have lost your own home, you can still have the privacy of your own space.

Staff

In May 2013 the then health minister in England announced that it was unacceptable that there were no clear government standards for the training that must take place in a care home. Research in the United States by Dr Roxanne Johnson had already demonstrated that the training required for dog groomers and hairdressers was more demanding than that required for care workers in some places. There may have been no government standards but very many care homes do have their own high standards. Particularly in the independent for profit sector, managers are aware that staff training has three distinct and money-saving advantages. First, it reduces staff turnover by improving staff morale, and staff turnover is rather expensive. Second, it reduces adverse incidents, which are damaging both financially and for reputational reasons, because old people get hurt and the complaints and aftermath are time-consuming. And third, it improves standards of care, which is good for business, because good care homes are at a premium and filling those beds is what keeps the business healthy. So even if operators have a heart of stone, enlightened self-interest makes them inclined to take advantage of some of the low-cost and free dementia education that is available. Large care home groups often have in-house trainers.

Ask what education people have had. It is more impressive if the training is from a reputable provider such as a university, or if it is accredited by an external organisation. However, note that degrees are useful for imparting knowledge but don't always automatically change practice in care homes. There is research in hospital care that suggests you are more likely to survive if your nurse has a degree, so it depends on what you are looking for. Don't be impressed by computerised courses for frontline staff. The most important element in improving care is the face-to-face teaching that imparts moral standards and personal values, in addition to the practical hands-on skills that are vital for the job. Staff learn how to talk to people with dementia by example from their leaders, who set the tone and standards for the place. It is really important, however, that someone on the team has a formal dementia qualification. There was a time when such qualifications were rare, and just being kind and doing your best were better than nothing. That's history. Staff need to have national vocational qualifications that are set down from time to time by government or other national agencies. However, they also need to know a lot about dementia, which is not always a regulatory requirement. You need to ask.

The core staff of a good home must include people with responsibility for social and recreational activity, cooks, grounds staff, housekeeping staff, drivers and administrators, and all of these should have dementia training as well. In addition to the core staff you would expect some or all of the following (and maybe others too) to be available at regular intervals and on call as required:

◆ barber, hairdresser and/or beautician;
◆ dementia liaison nurse or community psychiatric nurse;
◆ dentist;
◆ faith leaders for all faiths – chaplain, priest, rabbi, pastor, imam, preacher, minister;

◆ general practitioner;
◆ librarian or mobile library;
◆ local befrienders;
◆ masseur and/or exercise leader;
◆ musician and/or art therapist;
◆ occupational therapist, physiotherapist and/or dietician;
◆ optometrist;
◆ pet therapist;
◆ podiatrist;
◆ psychiatrist of old age;
◆ social worker.

My favourite care home has a twice-weekly visit from the ice cream van, complete with music. So I'd put that on the list as well.

Funding

Funding of care, whether in a person's own home or a residential or nursing home, is complicated. Getting information can be difficult and the rules can be hard to understand. In the past they were applied differently in different parts of the country. The process of applying is time-consuming and often bewildering. (Alzheimer's Society)

The system of payment for care homes is often seen as unfair, because people who worked and saved have to pay and people with no resources get support. Thinking about how you are going to fund this in future is crucial, and you can assume prices will not fall. Care homes that provide nursing care are generally more expensive than care homes that provide only residential care. The latest information on benefits needs to be sought, along with information about the person's current financial position, in order to work out what you are able to do. There are useful organisations that can help, in addition to the support that's available from social workers. When looking at information on the Internet, be sure that it applies to where you are living, as countries, states and provinces differ from each other.

In general, in the UK if you've got more than between £23,000 and £24,000 in assets you will have to fund all or part of your care. If you've got less money you may still have to make a contribution. When I was training to be a nurse in the last quarter of the twentieth century, all older people who needed looking after were in free long stay hospital beds. By the time I was a ward manager, my job was to move as many of those old people as possible into the new care homes that were emerging, where care was more homely, but still paid for by the government. Now the hospitals are discharging old people as fast as they can, but the person with dementia must pay from their own assets if they have any. This transition is a result of the rising number of people who need care, and a reduction in the number of working people able to pay taxes to support them.

In the United States, the cost of dementia care varies. Memory care requires a larger staff-to-resident ratio and additional training to ensure the safety of all the residents, therefore the cost is usually higher than other communities. Costs may vary, depending on the following factors:

- Level of care needed
- Size of room
- Whether a room is private or semi-private
- Geographical location of the community

According to Genworth.com, in 2012, the U.S. national average cost of memory care for a single resident was almost $5,000 a month. This cost does vary widely by care facility, however. For example, some communities were as low as $1,500 per month and other communities as high as $7,000 per month. (A Place for Mom)

At some point the vast majority of older Americans are going to need care, and health insurance and Medicare don't always cover what you want. You need to decide what you will want in future and then explore that. There are fifty states in the United States, each with different policies on this. Here is what is said in Minnesota:

Own Your Future aims to make Minnesotans aware of the importance of planning now to identify personal and financial options to meet their future long-term needs and to increase the number of Minnesotans who have taken action to address and provide for their future long-term needs.

Understanding health insurance requirements and costs is highly complex, and the law changes over time. AARP has an excellent web resource called The Health Care Law and You that offers a drop-down menu where you can check the situation in your own state or territory. www.healthlawanswers.aarp.org

A Place for Mom is 'the largest senior living referral service in the US and Canada'. It is significant that the process of finding the right place is so complicated that an agency such as this is kept busy. Other agencies also exist.

It's not possible to say how long you will stay in a care home. The average length of stay has been dropping, not least because people can't afford it for long and even local authorities can't afford care home places as easily as they used to. If you are relying on savings, you need to be sure that you've got enough to last your lifetime. You could sell your home and buy an annuity. That's a financial product where you pay a lump sum to an insurance company. They are betting that you die before you've had all the money back. You would then have paid more than you needed, but at least you would never have had to worry about the money running out. An equity-release scheme lets you borrow money on the value of your house. That money could theoretically run out.

There are organisations that will help you to appeal against decisions if you are unhappy. The funding situation is so important and changeable that you must not rely on any information in a book such as this or a printed leaflet. Find out directly what the situation is now from a reputable advisory organisation.

You may need to unpick some complex issues depending on whether the support you are receiving is classed as 'nursing' or 'social' care. Once again, get up-to-date information and advice from a reputable source. Useful names are suggested at the end of the book. Not least, you need to be clear what is included in the fees that are being paid in the home and what is extra, such as laundry or outings.

Aging populations are an issue across the world and though the immediate responses vary, all are headed in the same direction, away from government-funded aid towards more family and personal responsibility. In Australia, residential care is provided by a variety of organisations, including state governments, private operators and charitable organisations that are subsidised and regulated by the federal government. What governments can afford to do depends on their economic status and a range of demographic issues. In China, changing demographics as a result of the one child policy and increased physical health of the aging population means that care of older relatives is changing fast. The very recent model of keeping people at home means that Chinese families may not be accustomed to or like the idea of a care home, and central government regulation of such facilities that would protect old people is in its infancy so they might not all be very attractive. However, if one married couple were caring for four parents and eight grandparents, this would be hard to do without hired help. In addition to nursing homes set up by the government, several privately owned nursing homes have been set up in cities such as Beijing and Shanghai.

Although Germany has a range of interesting models of community care, care home use is high – about

40 per cent of people with moderate to severe dementia are institutionalised. The majority of patients in nursing homes do not receive special care programmes. A long term insurance law was established in 1994 to alleviate the huge cost of care for older people and it has continued to develop in that country.

People often ask me which is the best country in the world to have dementia, and the wide variation in costs and services makes this hard to say. India has few residential care facilities. Home based care by relatives is the norm, but this will change with changing families. The role of ARDSI (Alzheimer's and Related Disorders Society of India) is vital because many families do not have the skills to care for dementia and it makes life harder for both them and the person with dementia. In Europe people sometimes talk sentimentally about the days when families 'took care of their own'. The role of women in those families and societies is examined in new research described in chapter 14, Afterword. A well-managed residential facility may be the ideal solution to this stage of life, when the person can no longer stay alone at home. In the 'good old days' there were not so many people with dementia for a family to look after, because people died younger, often before dementia caught up with them and women were not able to go out to work.

Every society is different. In Hungary many old people still live close to their relatives, and are not dependent on automobiles, so some of the things that bother older people in the United States are not yet an issue there. Until recently people with severe dementia symptoms were housed in psychiatric hospitals but new legislation shifted this to nursing homes, and now most of them have waiting lists. In Poland there is a lack of specific services for dementia, but there is care in settings controlled by the Ministry of Health and Welfare. There is a large number of private welfare homes, but costs are very high, and they lack effective scrutiny.

The Netherlands is the only country to develop a separate nursing home medical discipline. The Dutch large-scale residential and nursing home facilities were designed more than 35 years ago. Japan has highly developed care services for people with dementia. Through long-term care insurance or health insurance, people can access residential care services, in specialist centres. Many providers are from the private sector. So I'd like to go to a Japanese planned care home, with a Dutch physician, with a Californian climate near Scotland. Or maybe Scandinavia, if the taxes were lower and there was more daylight in winter. I'm not sure I can make all of that work, so I will just try to stay fit and avoid having to go in a care home if humanly possible.

Choosing the right place

It is essential to visit and see for yourself. Only if this is completely impossible should you delegate the job to a trusted friend or other family member. You can speak to a family doctor or GP and ask local people about what they have experienced. Call associations such as those listed in the Alzheimer's Disease International website to see who can help you in your own country. Some solicitors offer a private 'social work' service to private clients.

I was on a one-year placement in New Zealand when my mother's dementia got so bad that she could not stay at home any longer. Her solicitor arranged for an experienced staff member to accompany her to visit a couple of recommended care homes and they negotiated a place, then helped to sell the house contents and put the house on the market. They kept up the visiting until I returned. (Caroline, daughter of woman with dementia in Scotland)

The quality and standards of care provision in care homes are monitored and inspected by regulators in each of the four UK countries, and residents in care homes have rights. The following relates to England:

The Care Quality Commission (CQC) is the regulator of health and social care in England, whether it's provided by the NHS, local authorities, private companies or voluntary organisations.

Under existing rules, independent healthcare and adult social services should be registered with the CQC. NHS providers, such as hospitals and ambulance services, must also be registered. Registration of organisations reassures the public when they receive a care service or treatment. It also enables the CQC to check that organisations are continuing to meet CQC standards.

The standards set out the quality of care and facilities that you should expect from a care provider. As a resident in a care home, you should expect:

◆ *The right to be treated politely and with dignity.*

◆ *The right to privacy for yourself, and your relatives and friends when they visit.*

◆ *The right to deal with your own finances and spend your money how you choose.*

◆ *The right to eat food that's prepared in line with your faith and to worship when and where you want to.*

◆ *The right to choose the food that you eat, and to be given the time and space to relax and enjoy your meal.*

◆ *The right to choose when you get up in the mornings and go to bed at night.*

◆ *The right to complain if you're unhappy with your care.*

The National Minimum Standards for care homes are outlined on the CQC website.

These standards are not enforceable by law, but the CQC can enforce fines, public warnings or close or suspend a service if they believe that people's basic rights or safety are at risk. Organisations that are closed or suspended are given the chance to meet the safety requirements and resume their service. (www.nhs.uk/CarersDirect/guide/practicalsupport/Pages/Carehomes.aspx).

Check out the regulatory standards where you are, and if none are published, you can use those from another place such as England as a sense check about what you can reasonably ask for and expect. For example in the United States, state governments oversee the licensing of nursing homes. Australia has the Australian Aged Care Quality Agency. Some countries do not yet have an oversight system like this.

You may not want to imagine potential problems, but it is worth getting confirmation of what will happen if the resident's condition deteriorates. Find out how much notice is given if they are required to leave and how much notice you have to give if you want to take them somewhere else. There is often more than one level of residential care. In some places this is called high and low, or residential and nursing. There is a difference between what each level is prepared to do. Residential homes might only provide help with washing, dressing and medication, going to the toilet, bathing and eating. Some have specialist training in dementia care. Nursing homes or more specialist units might have a qualified nurse on duty twenty-four hours a day and the care they provide is not just about dementia but also other illnesses and disabilities. Not all care homes are suitable for dementia and some are intolerant of a number of the behavioural disturbances that may come with dementia. Research shows that difficult behaviour in residents is frequently caused by the behaviour of the care workers and the design of the home, so it is galling if the home itself has caused the problem that the home is not prepared to tolerate. But you still need a plan for such a situation.

A care home is suitable if it can meet the needs of the person, the cost is right and there is an available place. The home must also be willing. Moving to another home or a less pleasing room within a home is disturbing for a resident with dementia. If the worst happens and you feel that the money is running out, you need to talk to someone as early as possible to get the resident assessed again to see if they are eligible for any more help.

Once the person has taken up residence

Everyone said what a relief it must be for me when Mum went in the home, but it was just a different sort of stress. I could not believe that they would look after her properly, or understand her little ways. I cried myself to sleep every night. (H.L., daughter)

A good care home will appreciate it if you take an active role when you come to visit. What do you want to do? Take your mum for a bath or a stroll outside. Help go through her wardrobe sorting out minor repairs or items that need to be replaced. Sew name tags in her clothes and talk to her and sing. Have your supper with her in her room.

I did not like the way they did her hair, all brushed back in a band. She didn't even look like my mum any more. (H.L., daughter)

You can tell the home what you want. Provide a photograph of how she has always worn her hair. Talk to the hairdresser and her key worker. They should be glad to make a relationship with you. You can advise and ask for change.

The perfect care home

It has been described as being like a fine hotel with good housekeeping, a great restaurant and superior entertainment. Anyone who has to stay in hotels a lot will tell you that the charm soon wears off. You start to long for a place that feels like home, where you can do what you want. You wouldn't have to rush down for breakfast in case the buffet is closed. You wouldn't have to dress up. You could invite your friends round, or keep your dog with you, and you could stick things on the walls and make changes in your own space. You sometimes might not want to go to the dining room but just have beans on toast in front of the TV. Anyone who has to stay in hotels will tell you that the entertainment is for the lowest common denominator of the guests, and that's not you. The perfect care home is different for each of us. One person might like to socialise, while another might prefer to be alone. One might be glad to watch sport on TV all day, while another might need the peace and quiet of a garden. One might want to rest and another to be busy. The perfect care home for each of us is the one that allows us to do what we want.

And what about the end? I want to die with dignity if I can. I don't want to make a fuss or cause trouble. Please don't haul me about and drag me into and out of baths and talk about me as if I'm not there. Don't make me go to hospital right at the end if you can keep me comfortable in the home. But before all that happens, can we just try to have a little fun and laughter? I will if you will.

chapter 12

The dangers of a hospital admission and how to avoid them

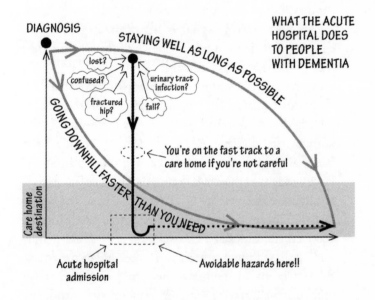

DIAGNOSIS

WHAT THE ACUTE HOSPITAL DOES TO PEOPLE WITH DEMENTIA

STAYING WELL AS LONG AS POSSIBLE

lost?

confused?

urinary tract infection?

fractured hip?

fall?

GOING DOWNHILL FASTER THAN YOU NEED

You're on the fast track to a care home if you're not careful

Care home destination

Acute hospital admission

Avoidable hazards here!!

People with dementia go into acute-care general hospitals more often than the rest of the population, even though acute-care hospitals are run as if every patient has perfect cognitive function. It is worth knowing how to help patients with dementia to avoid admission and what to do if your relative with dementia has to be in hospital. This is really important, because an acute hospital episode is full of avoidable dangers and can wreck stability for a person with dementia, causing chaos and distress for the rest of their life. You can be proactive to reduce these risks for your own loved ones (while others work on making hospitals safer for everyone). This chapter should help you with the emergency room (ER), guerrilla visiting tactics, reducing the risk of pain and delirium, how to look out for medication errors, and how to get out.

An acute-care hospital is like a meat grinder for people with dementia – it chews them up and spits them out – so well-run health systems are doing what they can to avoid admitting old people to hospital.

In Australia in 2013 nearly half of those patients who had dementia had no diagnosis before they were admitted to hospital. They would have come to the hospital with a range of problems, but without the knowledge that they had dementia on top of that, they would have been rather vulnerable. Toronto in Canada has a 'House Calls Programme' that has radically reduced the number of hospital visits for old people and increased the number who were able to die peacefully at home in their own bed. In the United States and Australia, having nursing staff on site in nursing homes has reduced the amount of hospital admissions that have been needed. Canadian data indicate that most people with dementia discharged after a period in hospital come out in a worse state than they went in. This is in line with what families and nursing home managers will tell you anecdotally. In Ontario they have GEM nurses in the emergency room – Geriatric Emergency Management nurses – who work to make it possible for the person to go home. There, as in other parts of the developed world, the patient with dementia when compared with another patient is two or three times more likely to be admitted to hospital and will stay two or three times as long. Apart from the discomfort, this costs a lot of money.

There is a lot you can do if your relative with dementia is in hospital. Your local acute general hospital might be one that has really prepared itself to welcome people with dementia. It would be wise to do so, as up to 50 per cent of patients may be either people with dementia or people with delirium, which looks similar and needs the same sort of response from staff. If this is the case, treat the rest of this chapter as of academic interest. And send me the name of your hospital, as I'd like to live near there.

The way we think about hospitals has evolved over time. What was an expensive luxury for our great-grandparents is now regarded as a routine service. A building that was once regarded with fear because so many people died there is now seen as desirable. We campaign against local hospital closures. We sometimes go there in preference to going to see our GP or primary care physician, as if the hospital was somehow superior and higher up the scale of effectiveness for all our ailments.

For people with dementia, nothing could be further from the truth. If they can stay out of hospital, so much the better. Of course, there are conditions which cannot be managed outside a hospital, but for many old people with dementia, getting admitted to hospital is the beginning of a slippery slope. They may have been managing perfectly well at home, but during their hospital stay things will happen that make them so unwell they never go home again. Research shows that if you have dementia you will stay in hospital longer than other people with the same clinical problem. For example, patients with dementia and a fractured hip tend not to be given as much pain relief as other patients with fractured hips. Uncontrolled pain in dementia gives rise to delirium that is often undiagnosed and untreated in hospitals. As a result, half of these patients die in six months.

There are many examples of people with dementia going hungry and thirsty in hospital. Patients with dementia may get missed by accident at mealtimes:

When James went to hospital I tried to get in at mealtimes to feed him, but visiting out of normal times was not allowed. He kept saying he was hungry, but they dismissed this as the dementia. After a couple of days I asked why it said 'nil by mouth' above his bed, and it turned out this notice was there from the last patient and they'd forgotten to take it down. He'd not eaten for days, and they'd ignored his pleas for food. (Wife of man with dementia)

From the outside, it sometimes looks as if the person had a crisis, had to go to hospital and then it was discovered that they weren't coping. In fact, it is often just the reverse. The person who was feeding themselves adequately will for a variety of reasons not get enough to eat in hospital. The person who was managing their own hygiene will not be able to negotiate the complexities and confusion of a hospital and will start to wet themselves and be unable to stay clean. This same person who managed to be happy and live quietly at home, sleeping at night and entertaining themselves by day, will be kept awake by noise and light at night, and bored to death in the daytime, never even seeing daylight. After a few days of that they'll become noisy and irritable and may be given medication to quieten them down. It is not unusual after this to have a fall or a fracture, leading to more surgery, and a long period in hospital during which all their skills leave them as they get undiagnosed depression and delirium, which at times is ignored by hospital staff and goes untreated, leading to early death.

I always say, if your mother is admitted to hospital, drop everything and go there. (Jan, dementia nurse specialist)

Delirium

Although delirium creates such a lot of problems, it is one of the least well-diagnosed and treated conditions in our hospitals. A list recently compiled by the president of the European Delirium Association includes about ten informal words that are used in medical notes referring to patients, such as 'knocked off', 'confused' and 'flat', which are not clinical terms but almost certainly indicate 'delirium'. In the same paper he gives some pseudo-scientific terms, such as 'acute brain failure' or 'acute confusional state', which also almost certainly suggest delirium. There is a proper treatment process for delirium and the condition is reversible, but there is no treatment for being 'confused', 'flat' or any of the other made-up descriptions. As a result of that misnaming or even absence of naming, the patient goes untreated even though their symptoms have been described in the notes. For a person with dementia, delirium can be fatal.

When I asked the nurse how my mother was, he said, 'Confused, as usual.' I asked him what it was about her behavior that was unexpected. He looked startled, not having expected further discussion and not realizing that I teach this subject to nurses. 'She doesn't do what I ask her,' he replied. He just assumed, because she is old, that this was normal for her, rather than a temporary clinical condition that he should be working to reverse using oxygen and plenty of drinks of water, and careful reassurance. (Dementia nurse teacher)

Of course, this is a terrible human story. And it's terrible financially too. If the person with dementia stays longer in hospital than others with the same condition it delays everyone else's treatment. The social services get handed back an old lady who needs a care home place, when what they had before was a semi-independent old lady who mainly looked after herself with a bit of home care. The family, if there is one, and the estate of the old lady now face the probability of having their assets stripped to pay for a situation that may have been avoidable.

People with dementia can avoid hospital in the first place by using all the advice in this book on how to live well with dementia (Chapters 6–10). Adapting the house and adopting some lifestyle changes can really make a difference. Note that the commonest reason for admission is a fall or a urinary tract infection. There is advice that will help you to reduce the risk of falling in Chapter 9. To be well you need a combination of diet, exposure to daylight, making enough use of light in the house, decluttering, choosing the right footwear and floor coverings, and exercise. In addition, avoiding urine infections is about making sure you drink lots of water.

In hospital, if the staff know what they are doing when they treat delirium, this ought to include:

◆ Hydration: the person needs to drink plenty.

◆ Oxygen: this is the fuel for the brain, so extra may be needed. It is tricky to get a person to keep a mask on when they are confused and upset, so you need to stay with them and help.

◆ Treating the underlying cause: delirium may be the result of medication they are on or an infection. It can also be brought on by stress in a person who is already compromised by mild cognitive impairment.

◆ Reassurance: delirium is terrifying and survivors may suffer from post-traumatic stress disorder, the psychological problem that affects people who have been in a war zone or a terrible accident, like a train crash.

When she got home my mother was reluctant to speak about it, but eventually she confessed that she had been certain that she had been taken to the intensive care unit to be euthanised. (Dementia nurse specialist)

Admission to hospital

Suppose you are arriving at the hospital with your elderly confused father. Here are the basics of surviving hospital for people with dementia and their caregivers.

First, don't leave him alone in the Emergency department. He could be there for ages and it is worth taking time off your work to be with him. Acting now could save you money and time in the long run. It means that you can make sure he gets to the bathroom and has a drink or whatever he needs to keep him well. Keep him warm if you find yourself in a draughty location like a corridor, and entertain and encourage him. At times you may also need to help him to stay cool, but remember that if he's immobile it probably feels cooler to him than to you or to the staff who are racing around. You can make sure his medication does not get missed. Hospitals are supposed to check 'cognitive status' (which means how well the patient's brain is working) on admission, but they often don't. In some cases even if they see a problem they don't take the right corrective measures anyway. If they did a careful examination they'd almost certainly know this patient has dementia or a related problem. There is a significant possibility that they won't notice it. You should tell them. You may have to mention it a number of times, because the staff member you tell sometimes does not understand the importance of what you are saying and does not write it down or communicate it. Have a notebook and a watch. At first they may say that he is not allowed to eat or drink until seen by the doctor. Pester them. Not drinking enough can make dementia much worse. Use words like 'dehydration' and 'delirium'. Smile.

Second, if the doctors or nurses say that they are going to admit him to hospital for 'assessment', check your watch. At the time of writing there is a national standard in Scotland that says patients must not be kept in the Emergency department for more than four hours. So if it is three hours and fifty minutes since you arrived, you have to make sure they are not admitting your relative to hospital because they ran out of the time they are allowed to keep him at the 'front door'. Tell them you don't mind if they breach their waiting time target if it means that you can take him home today. The danger is that they might be moving him into a danger zone for a reason that is more to do with their administrative pressures than his welfare. (This is always easier to argue if you have welfare power of attorney: see Chapter 13.)

The doctor said, 'We say to relatives that we've decided to admit the patient.' He added that if he was telling the truth he'd say, 'We've admitted to decide. That four-hour window does not give us enough time to know what we need to do, so we just bring them in, in case, and make up our minds later.' (Relative of man with dementia)

This means that you are being admitted to hospital in

case you've got something wrong that needs hospital admission rather than because the doctors really think you've got something that needs it. For most of us this might be inconvenient, scary or even entertaining. If you have dementia and the admission was not really necessary the consequences may be tragic.

Third, consider having some soft headphones and nice music or a story disc with you. The noise and turmoil in ER and the rest of the hospital will make him think he has died and gone to hell. Whatever he likes to listen to, on headphones, will reduce his stress and anxiety, and he can shut his eyes, knowing you are there. Touch him as much as you can, holding hands or stroking his hair. It will make him feel better and the staff will notice. Keep yourself hydrated and your blood sugar up, stay alert and keep good eye contact with staff.

Fourth, don't leave your father – especially when staff ask you to. I hear tales of caregivers who are sent from the cubicle when people with dementia are examined by medics on the grounds of confidentiality. This is silly. The person with dementia needs someone consistent to know what is going on. Even if you don't have a legal document, no court is going to send you to jail for insisting on protecting a vulnerable adult. Let the doctor or nurse carry out their examination and let your relative do all the answering that he is going to do. If he speaks for himself and says the wrong thing, don't interrupt. They need to hear him saying the wrong thing or being slow, or not replying. Wait until you are asked or until the end of the examination to point out that he does not live where he said he lives any more, or that his age is different from what he said, or to fill in the blanks. Also, make sure they know if he is much worse than usual. Sometimes they assume that because a patient has dementia, how confused they are in ER is 'baseline normal' for the patient. If it is not, make sure that clinical staff know this. If he's more confused than usual there will almost certainly be a reversible cause, and that is what the hospital needs to focus on and reverse.

The reason for unnecessary hospital admissions of people with dementia seems to be related to hospital staff not having much experience of people with this condition, with the result that they can't believe that the person is going to survive a night at home. In addition, the hospital doctor may have anxieties that if the person they are sending home has an adverse outcome subsequently, they will be held personally responsible. Interestingly, if it turns out that the hospital admission has a bad outcome that does not seem to worry the admitting doctor or give rise to questions about standards of care. Go home and fall = my fault. Go into hospital and fall = the system's responsibility. This is how the system makes clinicians think, even when risk of an accident or adverse incident in hospital is higher. Research shows that people with dementia in hospital are more likely to have falls and other adverse incidents:

My husband was in a side room on his own and he kept trying to get out of bed. Because of his dementia he was unsteady on his feet and confused and anxious. They were worried about him being incontinent. I said, 'Please don't put a catheter in – he'll only pull it out and hurt himself. I'll stay the night with him.' But they sent me home. It wasn't allowed for me to stay. That night he did pull the catheter out and then he fell on the floor climbing over the cot sides they put on his bed to try to contain him. (Widow of 72-year-old man with dementia)

Many hospitals have brave and clever plans to overcome this perverse incentive to admit patients, including rapid-response teams and specialist nurses, but it is a serious issue that continues to cause concern. You need to keep an eye out for your relative.

It might turn out that there is something wrong that absolutely requires a hospital stay. Some hospitals are geared up for this, having a system called the 'Blue Butterfly' scheme or something similar that means staff are alerted to the presence of a person with dementia and know how to support them by discreetly identifying them with a little sign on their notes or by the bedside. They should ask you or the patient if they mind being identified in this way, as technically this would be disclosing the diagnosis to people who theoretically might not need to know. Be assured, if the patient has dementia, everyone needs to know, including domestic staff and administrators. If staff see the butterfly sign, they know what to do differently for that patient. Hydrate. Explain yourself. Repeat yourself. Keep the atmosphere calm. In fact, all the strategies covered in Chapter 7 about how to understand and manage disturbing behaviours at home should be followed in hospital.

Of course, it won't work unless staff are educated about what will make a person with dementia worse. I've seen people with dementia hurtled through a busy hospital to their destination ward on their back on a trolley by porters or other staff chatting to each other or using cellphones or radios. It's a nightmare. People with dementia are incredibly stressed already, so why would health workers do something to make things worse? If your relative is in a bad hospital, you can't change that hospital, but your presence may improve or modify the behaviour of some of the staff. Sometimes it is not just carelessness but not knowing what is needed.

The referring doctor may already have made a careful and correct assessment that the person needs to be in hospital. Even so, the hospital is sometimes organised in a way that means they can't go straight to a bed when they get there, but have to pass through the ER and all the assessment processes as if they had just come in off the street, even though the primary care clinician who knows them well has already done the assessment. The patient then has to bend to their systems, even though they have already been classified by an experienced doctor as fragile. Be ready to protect them.

My dad was told he was going to the hospital for assessment, but when he got there different people kept asking him why he had come and what was wrong. We waited for hours for the doctors. When they arrived, they pulled the drapes round and indicated I was to go away. When I saw Dad again he had no idea what had happened or been decided and no one told me, even though I told them he had dementia and I am his caregiver. (Daughter of J.G.)

When a patient arrives on a hospital ward there are some procedures that ought to happen if the patient is known to have dementia, but also arrangements including specific design elements should be in place to make them comfortable.

The patient with dementia should be nursed in a single, not shared, room if possible to minimise noise and disturbance. People with dementia find it hard to make sense of what they are hearing, so background noise is a greater problem for them than other people. It gets in the way of understanding what people are saying to them, or concentrating on essential tasks like eating. The chaos that can be caused by a person with dementia can agitate everyone else and set other patients off into angry or disturbing behaviour, so you can help staff understand that a single room is not a privilege for your mum or dad, but offers advantages for their fellow patients. The controlled environment will make it less likely that his or her behaviour will become disturbing, particularly as family and friends will find it easier to stay and keep them company. It will also be easier to keep the place quiet and dark at night, helping them to sleep. If the curtains don't fit the window, that's going to be a problem for any patient who is accustomed to sleeping in the dark. A window in the door is particularly unhelpful. The patient then sees confusing moving pictures in the night and will be inclined to get out of bed to investigate. Nurses say they like it for observation, but if that was important they could prop the door open. You can't change the design, but if you are aware of these common misperceptions that people with dementia get, you can help explain his or her behaviour to the staff and that might prevent some inappropriate staff responses:

The ward sister said to me, 'We can't make a fuss of her just because you say she's got dementia. I've got everyone else to think about.' I was so disheartened that I could not argue. I wanted to tell her that I WAS thinking about everyone else. Mum's behavior is so embarrassing. You hear the other patients complaining to their visitors. But when she got moved to a side room it was much easier for her and everyone else, and I was able to stay overnight with her. (Daughter of Ethel, 90)

The room should have an ensuite shower room because getting to and from the toilet is fraught with hazards for people with dementia. In a strange environment they can't remember what they've been told about where it is. Having your own is ideal, in particular if the door is open and there is good signage. Experts talk about 'architectural incontinence'. That's when the person wets themselves because the building was designed in such a way that they could not find the bathroom in time. All the elements that were described in Chapter 9 would help. Even though you can't improve the design of the room in the short time you are there, if you are aware of the limitations of the design you can work with them.

The room needs to be well lit in the daytime. There

should be a window that at least shows what time of day it is by allowing daylight in, and some vegetation or a view outside makes a real difference. Exposure to daylight affects the body clock even more in old people with dementia, so it would be brilliant if there was access to an outside garden or terrace in daylight hours, especially the morning.

Our hospital has a lovely courtyard garden that you can see through the windows, but the doors are locked and no one can walk in there. (Hospital manager)

From the bed there should be a visible clock, and a calendar would be useful. If there is a metal flip-top bin the lid should be fitted with a dampener, to stop it clanging every time a doctor washes her hands and throws in a paper towel. It is possible to be prescriptive about these things in a hospital, because statistics show that every hospital room is going to have a person with dementia or cognitive impairment in it at some point. Up to 50 per cent of patients are affected. In chapter 9, on home design modifications, the advice is less prescriptive because you don't want to change too many familiar elements at home. In a hospital it is inexcusable to fail to provide evidence-based dementia-friendly design and fittings. There is a limit to how much you can modify a room when it has been allocated, but if it does not have the right design features, be sure to complain to the hospital afterwards, in writing. Recommend to them the free dementia-friendly hospital design guidance on the Internet (www.dementia.stir.ac.uk/design/virtual-environments/virtual-hospital) and point out that many of the changes are low-cost and will pay for themselves in a very short time, by the reduction of adverse incidents and accidents, like falls.

Hospital floor surfaces are often shiny and reflective. Because this makes them look wet, and people with dementia may have problems with depth perception and visual impairment, they'll be uncertain about walking on those potentially icy or slippery surfaces and might fall over as a result. It is really helpful if the environment is uncluttered. Hospitals have too many pointless signs and out-of-date notices and not enough attention is paid to essential information and way-finding needs. Bathrooms are frequently stark in their decoration, but also used as an equipment store and location for extra boxes of supplies. A person with dementia being taken for a bath there would be justified in wondering what was happening if asked to undress in that environment. If your relative starts to show disturbing behaviour in this environment, you can point out the problems to the staff.

My mother does not like showers and she hated having her bath in hospital and so I went in and did it myself. We had fun, and it was relaxing for her. But I had to drape some sheets over the junk in the room to make it more homely for her. (Daughter of Keesha, 83)

Often staff will inform patients about the nurse call system. Ideally this should be a silent one involving vibrating pagers, so that the patient does not have to listen to buzzers going off all day and night or put up with flashing lights. These have been available for some time, but they are still rare for no other reason than that staff don't ask for them and maintenance departments haven't been persuaded to fit them. Of course, if you've got dementia you won't remember what the nurse said, so you won't remember how to call. Movement sensors are easily available but not often used for this sort of patient. Hospitals do not fold round you when you have this sort of vulnerability.

Your relative should have access to plentiful supplies of fluids, unless he is on some special regimen that limits them. Be aware that the drinking jug is sometimes accidentally or carelessly placed out of reach by staff, and if it is made of clear plastic filled with clear water, and out of the line of sight, it might also be effectively invisible. People with dementia follow visual cues more than some others. Maybe squirt some orange in it, or put it nearer.

General issues about medication safety

Keep a close eye on the medication. Sometimes doctors need to take the patient off previous medication to see if that is what has been making them ill. But sometimes this is not well enough thought through. For example, the person with dementia might be used to managing their own medication and they might not comply with what is going on because they are not given an explanation at every medicine round and they forget or can't work out what is happening.

When I went to see Mum in hospital she said, 'Can I come

*home?' and I said, 'Not till they make you better, Mum,'
and she said, 'How're they going to do that, darling?'
and I said, 'They'll most likely give you pills, Mum,' and
she said, 'What? Like these?' And she took half a dozen
assorted capsules out of her dressing-gown pocket. She said,
'They've given me the wrong ones, so I've not been taking
them, and I didn't like to say they were wrong in case the
nurse got into trouble.' (Daughter of Dominka, 75)*

Being given the wrong medicine is a common hazard of
being in hospital. In this case it was the right medicine
but the patient was trying to protect herself against
being poisoned accidentally. She had dementia but she
was not stupid.

Sometimes hospitals decide to reduce the amount of
medication that the older person has been taking and
change it, but this can be really disruptive. Your reports
of what your relative was like previously are really
important. Because they are old, staff sometimes make
assumptions and have low expectations for the patient,
assuming they are headed for a care facility. Issues that
have arisen for the first time in this patient are not ques-
tioned. The assumption is that all old people or people
with dementia are like this.

*The painkillers that my mom has been taking have horrible
side effects, we know, but when she got to hospital they
took her right off them. The next day they said, 'Of course,
she's incontinent, and she's had a fall ...' and I was so
surprised because she never had been incontinent and they
had accepted it as normal for her. I realised she suddenly got
incontinent because the uncontrolled pain meant she could*

not move fast enough to get to their bathroom and had an accident on the way. She was so upset and ended up wetting on the floor and slipping in it. (Daughter of Temeeka, 73)

A second issue is that the person with dementia is frequently started on antipsychotic medication in hospital to keep them quiet. This is the term for a range of drugs that will sedate the patient when they are noisy and disruptive. Depending on what sort of dementia the person has this medication could finish them off (see Chapter 2). All medicine involves risk, and it might be that the person has to have antipsychotics as a last resort for some horribly severe and complex symptoms, but make sure that the doctors really are using them as a last resort and not just reaching for the first response they think of. Professor Sube Banerjee reported in 2013 that in the UK 180,000 old people were given antipsychotic medication every year, but less than a quarter of them got any real benefit, and about 1,800 old people die each year as a result of this particular medicine. If it was children dying there would be a riot. Our press is less sensitive to the death of older people, reflecting the values of our society. Just don't let it be your parent.

It is best practice for a hospital to start to plan the discharge of the patient the moment they arrive. The aim should be to return them home (or to their care home, if that is where they came from) with their medical problem resolved. There is evidence that hospital staff sometimes see an old person with dementia arriving from their own home, ill and dishevelled, and assume from the start that they are only ever going to be fit for a care facility. The outcome for the old person is determined and fixed by this assumption. To be fair, the tendency to delay discussion about 'what next?' and 'what if?' is endemic in families as well. How many of us have had the conversation with our own children about what we want to happen when we become frail, or if we lose capacity to make decisions? Do we want to be resuscitated and treated assertively? Do we mind going into a home? How much risk are we prepared to tolerate?

It is never too soon after an admission to hospital to start the family conversation about where the person will go. Unfortunately, many people with dementia languish in hospital for months after they are able to move on, simply because we have not got ourselves into gear from the start and planned what was going to happen next. The day to check out home care services is the day the person is admitted to hospital, not the day they are described as ready to go. It is even better if you thought about it last year.

Visiting

One day I was headed towards the door of a ward to give advice about a person with dementia who was creating difficulties for the staff only to be met by an irritated nurse who all but put the palm of her hand in my face and barked, 'No visitors till three.' Disconcerted, and in fact not quite sure if I'd heard right, I stepped back.

Behind me was an elderly man with a flat cap and a

small suitcase on his lap, sitting on a bench. He shook his head. 'You'll not get in till three, dearie,' he said. Glancing at my watch, I saw it was four minutes to three. So I sat beside him, even though I was meant to be working. He was desperate to get in. His wife of sixty years was in there in a terrible old nightdress that she was ashamed of and he had her nicest clothes in the bag. He'd been sitting for about half an hour, having arrived in good time with the clothes in the mistaken understanding that he'd be able to get them to her before visiting started. Dead on three the ward doors opened with a crash and the anxious relatives from the waiting area went through to make the best of the strictly limited access to their loved ones. It's not good. Staff were embarrassed about the hand in my face when they worked out who I was, but were clearly unconcerned about the personal issues for the lady or her husband. (Hospital visitor)

There is nothing you can be doing in hospital that cannot be interrupted by staff. When I was a ward sister I had to defend an elderly patient one day when the doctor arrived, wishing to undertake an examination which involved inserting a gloved finger in his bottom. The doctor had forgotten to do that part of the examination earlier and the gentleman was now sitting up eating his dinner. As it was not a life and death issue, I asked the doctor to return later, which was clearly not convenient for her. To be honest, we argued, and it got bitter, but in the end she agreed.

It is as if there is a perverse hierarchy of need. We need to keep the system working, then we need to satisfy the requirements of staff to undertake their ritualistic tasks, then we need to address routine issues and only then the 'ordinary' things, like sleeping, eating, having your loved ones beside you comforting and caring for you, and much more. These ordinary things are so far down the line and unimportant to staff that they sometimes get excluded. You can work to reverse that order for your relative.

As it happens, those are the things that make most difference to a person with dementia. Your dad is more likely to cooperate with the staff if you are with him offering reassurance. If they don't have time to wait for him to do slowly what you know he can do for himself, you may be able to take that off them and let them rush about helping other patients. The point is that they avoid doing very much to patients during visiting. At the one time of day when they let you in to visit, they usually don't create any opportunities for you to do useful activities like helping with changing clothes or with eating. They treat visiting time like my granny treated unfamiliar or posh visitors to her house; tidy up till they get here, then stop doing anything and give a good impression. Family visits should involve sprawling about and having treats and laughter. No impression is needed apart from love and fun and the eating of Jaffa Cakes or whatever your granny calls them. That is the sort of hospital visiting that would be perfect for a person with dementia.

Of course, there are limits, and it depends what's wrong with the person. But don't just sit there politely eyeing the grapes. Do something. My advice is, be a guerrilla visitor. Find ways of having open visiting if only for this patient. Challenge and defy the visiting times and rules. Make rotas with friends and family to make sure the person is not left to the mercy of the system.

Useful things to do while visiting:

◆ If possible, take the person with dementia for some exercise. It is one of the most important elements of dementia care (see Chapter 6, page 134). Very many people have their mobility vastly reduced as a result of a hospital stay.

◆ If possible, get them into daylight. This may mean commandeering a wheelchair, because although many hospitals have gardens, many are not easy to get to. You may have to insist on a key for access.

◆ Take as many personal objects – for example, cards from grandchildren, drawn pictures, photos, pot plants – as you think you can reasonably get away with and festoon their bed space. Patients who appear to have a large and interested family seem to get more attention, and objects demonstrate that. It's not a research-based observation but one can imagine why it is the case.

◆ Have a memory book or communications passport. This is often a scrapbook or notebook that allows you to record the person's likes and dislikes so there is no excuse for staff 'not knowing' when you aren't there. It is not fair to give the staff the responsibility of the only copy, so try to have multiples. Knowing more about the person with dementia helps the hospital workers to build relationships. The Alzheimer Society websites in many countries have local versions of a template for this, or you can borrow one from the Alzheimer Society of Canada which has produced one called 'All About Me'. Imitation is the sincerest form of flattery. They won't mind.

◆ Encourage eating and drinking. You need to check about any medical issues, but often there's no limit to what you can bring and they might well not be eating the hospital food. Find out what their heart's desire is. Ice cream? Belgian chocolate? Steak? Tripe à la mode de Caen? Then get it to them by hook or by crook.

◆ Check their ankles for swelling. If I had a pound for every old lady I find in hospital with swollen ankles, sitting up all day in a chair with her legs dangling, I'd be rich. Draw it to the attention of the staff and make sure they've got ways of keeping their feet up.

◆ Check their bony bits (and bum – you only need to ask) for redness and soreness. A person who does not move about enough, who is constipated and dehydrated and sometimes incontinent will get sore where the skin and bone are pressed together on their bottom or their heels and elbows. After the redness, the skin can break and become infected and this necrosis is called a pressure sore. Shamefully, they occur in people who are being 'cared for' in hospital.

◆ Take them to the bathroom and wash their hands.

◆ Insist on speaking to staff about their condition. If you have power of attorney (see Chapter 13) you can do quite a lot. Nursing staff may say that you need to talk to the doctor, who is not available, and that you will need to make an appointment. That's not good enough. Insist on reading the notes. That often results in a doctor being found.

◆ Find a way of letting the staff know 'who' is in the bed. Did this little man in the bed once blow up some tanks? Did he bake amazing bread? Does he have twenty-five grandchildren, one of whom is a sharp lawyer who specialises in medical negligence? (I once discovered a formerly terrifying matron languishing in a hospital bed and the nursing staff did not even know that this old lady had ever been a nurse, far less that she designed most of the training they'd had.)

Increasingly, we are trying to get hospital staff to see family and friends as extra pairs of hands. If they can visit at mealtimes and help to encourage the person to eat, and eat alongside them, that's good. If they can help by making sure the patient washes their hands before eating and after, and taking them to the toilet and helping with hygiene in the way they would at home, that is great too.

Bed moves can be fatal

Hospitals are under pressure to look after lots of patients as quickly as possible, because doing it slowly costs more money and there are always people having to wait in line for treatment or having procedures cancelled.

The design of most hospitals makes all of this even more difficult than it needs to be. Patients are often grouped in a 'bay' of four or six people. If they were all in single rooms it would be simple. When one patient in a single room has died or been moved, another could take his place. Because the majority of patients are in a bay, if one of the ladies dies or leaves, they need another female to take up the place. If the next patient in line waiting in the Emergency Department is a male – your dad, for example – it presents a practical problem. He can't go in with five ladies. He has to have a side room, because the only available bay space is 'female'. That's nice for him. But the lady who was in that side room has to be moved to the female bay to give him his space, and that can be very confusing for her if she has dementia. A day later, after he has settled in, they might need a man to make up a space in a male bay and release a side room for a lady – so out he goes. Dementia or not, he gets moved, even though there is research that shows it is very bad for people with dementia to be moved. Sometimes shuffling the spaces means that the patient has to go to another ward. For example, if the gynaecology ward, which deals with specific female problems and the ladies are mainly having surgery, has a vacant female bed, an old lady might get put there to make space for a man in the medical ward. These moves can take place at any time of day or night. Just imagine how it feels to wake from a drugged sleep and find yourself hurtling again along dimly lit hospital corridors, among strangers. It is a total pain if you've just worked out where the toilet is and now you've got to work all that stuff out again in a new ward.

You go to the bed where your mum was at the last

visiting time and the drapes are round a body covered in a sheet and people are talking in hushed whispers. Actually she's not dead, but the person who got her space is. She's on the terrace having a cup of tea. Not very funny. Or you arrive when the empty bed is being washed for the next person and the staff can't actually tell you very quickly where your mum is. And they say things like, 'She's gone', and your heart stops because she is a notorious wanderer and you think they've let her leave without telling you. And the ward clerk ruffling through the records laughs and says, 'Oh, I've lost her … Where's she gone? … I've just come back from vacation and I can't find anything …'

You might not think there's much you can do about the bed-move problem. It really does not help to get angry, because the nurses in front of you feel they have little control over the system. You can manage the situation and do what you can to make sure that, if anyone is disadvantaged, it's not your loved one. Other people are responsible for the system; you are only responsible for this one person. The fundamental plan is to make sure that they only move your person as a last resort, on the understanding that you will make a significant issue about it.

First, make sure that the hospital and ward have your contact details which work twenty-four hours a day. Pretend you don't have a landline. Don't give them a landline number, because if you don't answer at any time, they sometimes don't have a plan B for getting in touch with you.

I got to the hospital and Dad was dead. It was such a shock. It took me two hours to get there, and he had been dead for two hours. They said they called my home number and I had just left so they did not leave a message. My husband, who was in the house, could have called me on the cellphone. The nurses could have called me on the cell. But they had a policy of not calling cellphones. I was too distressed to drive and it took my husband hours to come to get to me to take me home. I sat and cried in the entrance. (Daughter of Jonathan, 79)

Second, make a special request to the staff that if there is any question of patients being moved, your dad should be a priority for staying put, particularly if he is lucky enough to be in a single room. Remind them that if he had an infectious disease they'd not move him out of isolation and that dementia is like an infectious disease. For example, if he is noisy at night in a bay of patients, no one else is going to get any sleep and other relatives will complain, apart from the effect it will have on staff and patients. His dementia would affect the well-being and recovery of others, and this could be prevented by keeping him in the side room. Specifically, ask them if they could mention this to the 'bed manager'. The bed manager is an overarching nurse who has the power to tell the staff in any ward to vacate beds or move the occupant to a different place – or to leave them where they are.

Third, if a bed move happens, step up your visiting and mention that you will consider making a formal complaint if it happens again, as you are aware that multiple moves pose an avoidable risk for people with dementia. You may wish to say that the only acceptable move would be into a single room, if they are not already in one.

Pain relief

There is research showing that when people with dementia in hospital are suffering pain they are less likely than other patients to be given something to help. The way you get medicines in hospitals is usually like this. First, they throw away all the pills that you've been on, prescribed by previous consultants and your family doctor. Then the hospital doctor examines you and writes a prescription for use during your admission. It's often on a big chart kept at the end of the bed. This might include any of the medicines that all the previous experts said you needed. With luck the hospital doctor will have stopped only those pills that were working against each other or not working at all. Very many older people are on five or more different medicines and it is highly likely that these are making the person more ill in some way. One problem is that if the hospital doctor prescribes something which is exactly what the person was taking at home, the hospital pharmacy may issue a different pill from a different manufacturer, so the colour or size looks different. It can be very confusing. The nurses are supposed to explain, but in practice I see little medicine pots of pills being popped down beside the breakfast tray. Leaving medicines with patients is often said to be a result of nurses being 'too busy'. Of course everyone is very busy, but this just offers opportunities for patients to put pills in their dressing-gown pocket or for other patients to inadvertently swallow them. And it is strictly against all nursing codes of practice. What does it say if hospital nurses are too busy to give patients the medicines that are meant to make them better?

The tablets, injections or intravenous drips that the hospital doctor prescribes can be given in two ways. The first is to administer the medication at regular intervals – for example, four times a day or twice a day. Sometimes the timing between pills is so important that the nurses will wake you up to give them to you. Sometimes the timing of medication can be more relaxed, and it is given at roughly breakfast, lunch, teatime and bedtime. And when the staff are busy it might be astonishingly early or late. Sometimes they just forget. The second way is that the medication is given on demand. Doctors write permission for this on the prescription chart using the letters 'PRN' or the words 'as required', only stating a limit to the number of doses. For example, you might be 'written up' for paracetamol 'for pain PRN up to four times a day'. In those cases, the nurse will come to you at the time she's giving out the other pills and say, 'Have you got pain?' and if you say yes, she'll give you paracetamol for it. If you say no, she'll perhaps ask you another time. Or you might get some in between medicine rounds if you actually complain of pain. Or not ever.

This is where the provision of pain relief to people with dementia in hospital falls down. If an old lady thinks she is at the golf club and someone in uniform looms up and asks such an odd question, she'll say, 'No', wondering why the 'waitress' has asked her this. Even if she was in pain she'd not tell them. Why should she? Often people with dementia say no at first to most suggestions. It is the safest answer if you are not sure what is going on and what they are going to do to you. This may explain why, in hip fracture cases, research shows that people with dementia get less post-operative pain relief than other patients of the same age with the same condition. In addition, many older people have some painful condition or other, like arthritis, which may get worse or feel worse in the unfamiliar routine and confines of hospital. Older people with dementia may be poor at communicating that they are in pain when asked, and may not understand the system that requires them to ask for pain relief between medicine rounds. It is better practice just to give routine pain-killers on a regular basis, or to give them a 'pain patch', which looks like a sticking plaster and is a transdermal preparation that slowly releases pain-relieving medicine through the skin over time.

If pain relief was a bad thing, frugality with the drugs would be a good thing. However, research shows that if a person with dementia suffers pain, they are very likely to get delirium. Delirium, as has been said, can be fatal, in addition to being deeply unpleasant. Rather than saying that they are in pain, people with dementia communicate their untreated pain by becoming agitated, or aggressive, or trying to leave the area. When I am consulted about disturbing behaviour in older people with dementia in hospital, my first question is routine pain relief. Sadly, many hospital workers might first reach for a sedative, like the dreaded antipsychotic medication, thus leaving the person with dementia still in pain but stupefied and wobbly on their feet.

I made the mistake of asking, 'Is my mother on any painkillers?' because she was so agitated, and they said, 'Oh, yes!' and rattled off the names from the prescription chart. I was at the front door when I had another thought and went back up to the ward and asked a second question. 'When did my mother last have a painkiller?' and the same nurse looked at the chart and said briskly, 'She's not had any for six days.' I had originally asked the wrong question. Who knew? When she was given some pain relief she started to calm down within thirty minutes. (Daughter of Alice, 96)

It is reasonable for you as a caregiver to ask the ward staff what 'pain scale' they use to assess whether a patient with dementia is in pain, and ask to see the results for your relative. A pain scale is a formal method of estimating how much a patient is in pain. It might include a diagram of a body so the patient can point to where it hurts. It may include a series of questions to help decide how much pain the person is suffering. You may have heard medics on TV in emergency programmes saying, 'On a scale of one to ten, how bad is the pain in your chest?' and the patient gasps out a number. Because people with dementia have communication difficulties and sometimes can't answer a question as clearly as that, there are special pain scales that are used in best practice to decide whether people with dementia are suffering pain and where it is, often using facial expression and movement as a guide. There is extensive research on pain in dementia patients and guidance available for staff on how to assess pain. Some painkillers that work well for most of us may cause problems for older people with dementia because when they are broken down by the liver they create substances that make delirium or other symptoms worse. It's a problem. They either don't give you pain relief or they dose you with something that is going to be bad for you. Guidance on how to do good pain control is available from professional organisations and you can check whether staff are adhering to the guidance by asking, for example, if they are using one of the recognised dementia pain scales (a famous one is the 'Abbey' pain scale). Ask to see what they are using.

The main danger to look out for is your relative being given sedation to stop them expressing their pain. To be bewildered and in agony is a nightmare.

Something to do

There is a further dilemma here. If acute hospitals were working properly, people with dementia who don't need hospital care would not be sitting in them for three months after they are ready to leave. On the other hand, because these waits are a reality, acute-care hospitals need to be providing an environment and stimulation that will help to maintain the person with dementia. It is quite reasonable to ask if you can bring the pet dog up to visit, even if the reunion has to take place in the hospital garden. You are justified in challenging the nursing staff if there is meaningless endless TV on which no one is watching. Jolly music is all very well, but no one wants it all the time (apart from some of the staff). Sometimes the hospital is happy for you to take their patient out for a trip home or for lunch, for example. Ask about a 'day pass', which is a formal agreement for you to take the patient away with a guarantee that the bed will be there when you get back. After all, if they have said your mother is ready for home, they can't detain her. Watch out for a tendency to overemphasise what she can't do, which would make her nervous about coming out and about with you, and make you nervous too. She might be their patient, but she's also your mum and a free citizen.

Just as I was leaving at the end of visiting, JP got me by the sleeve and begged me to get him out of there before he went mad. After two weeks he became passive and querulous, and afraid to come home with me. He told me that I'd not be able to cope because he said 'they say it takes two to lift me, and you can't do that…' (Daughter-in-law)

The simplest things can make a difference. Staff might arrange some chairs around a table so patients can sit in companionable silence looking at the paper and drinking tea, or they could begin to chat or start a game of poker – anything to relieve the boredom. Nurses often require everyone to be neat and tidy beside their bed, too far away from anyone else to talk, even in the bay with five other humans. You can help to make the place more sociable. If the hospital has volunteers or a chaplain, find them and let them know that your relative would welcome a visit. Make a donation to them in cash or kind. Buy attention, if you can afford to. Ask if you can pay for a visiting hairdresser to fix their hair or beautician to come and do a manicure. Give your dad a hot shave. Don't be afraid to take some control of the environment.

There were three daughters who used to take their mother for a bath at visiting time on our ward. She loved those visits, and came out all relaxed, cleaned and moisturised and ready for bed. In anticipation I used to clean the bathroom, and one day was just leaving it when they came in. Her daughter assured me that I did not need to because they brought their own cleaning materials and toiletries and cleaned our bathroom before and after bathing her. They had actually been put off by the poor level of the hospital's hygiene and were embarrassed to say it, so they were quietly protecting their mother, and replacing what would have been a staff chore with an act of well-organised tenderness. (Jane, 59)

The use of restraint

Make no mistake, relatives are the last people to create unnecessary fuss about the use of protective restraint. On the contrary, they are afraid that hospitals will fail to protect the person with dementia. There are practical reasons why one might restrain your mother during an admission to hospital. For example, she might be trying to get outside in her pyjamas, or trying to get into a man's bed in the next ward. General hospital patients here are not usually legally detained, and being restrained under those circumstances is a serious and potentially illegal deprivation of liberty. This is why the professional had better be sure that nothing goes wrong. If they take a risk and restrain someone, and no harm is done and no one complains, it might be OK. However, if something goes wrong they will be in serious trouble, and quite rightly so. The proper use of restraint requires them to involve families or others in discussion about its use, and it needs to be reviewed.

The problem with the use of restraint appears to be the extent to which staff fail to assess the underlying reason for the behaviour that is disturbing them. Research has been done on wandering that makes it clear that this walking behaviour is rational and not aimless. The person needs to walk about to try to clear their head, or check where they are, or relieve muscle stiffness, or get rid of tension. The worst thing you can do is try to restrict them to a chair when they feel like walking. This sometimes gives rise to frustration, anger and aggression, which may be followed by sedation, with all the problems that are associated with it, such as falls, disturbed sleep patterns and sometimes death.

Cot rails at the sides of beds are a particular problem. They are great if your bed is being moved rapidly and you might fall out. They are very bad if you are a person with dementia.

When I was in hospital there was a confused man in our bay. He kept getting out of bed and the nurses wanted him to stay there. The care assistant was in the bay at one point when he was about to get out. She put up the cot rails on either side of the bed and told him to stay put in no uncertain terms. After she'd gone he started shuffling to the end of the bed, determined to leave. The other guys in the other beds started shouting at him to lie down. Can you believe it? They thought they were helping the nurse by abusing the old fellow verbally. He kept shuffling and got his pyjama leg caught in the rail. Then he wet himself and cried. (Yalchin, 56)

In some hospitals cot rails are banned as a result of accidents where patients have managed to kill themselves when their head became trapped between the rail and the bed while trying to get out. If they climb over the top of the rail they may fall to the floor from an even greater height than if they just rolled off the bed. It is OK for you to object to a cot side. If they want your dad not to fall out of bed, they can offer a low-profile bed: that is, one that goes really low so he's only about a foot off the ground.

But physical restraint is not the only kind:

Last week I was in an NHS male hospital ward at about six in the evening and saw a room with eight or ten men all lying still in bed. Some were snoring noisily. It looked neat and peaceful to my colleague, but to me it looked like a Haloperidol party.* (Mark, hospital visitor)

If you think that restraint is being used you need to find

---

* Haloperidol is a frequently misused sedative for older people with dementia.

out what the problem was and whether they have tried other solutions. Hospitals are required to record that they are doing it and why, and to review it regularly. And you need to tell them that for best practice they should have consulted you before using it. It is most often used for disturbing behaviour and alternatives to restraint are described in Chapter 7. Check if they have tried those alternatives. The main danger is the redoubled efforts of the person with dementia to do what they were planning before the restraint was placed upon them.

Going home

Nothing defines an experience like the end of it, and the end of a hospital stay can be awful or wonderful. Official guidance on discharge from hospital usually emphasises that the aim should be to get the person back to their own previous environment. When you have dementia, even something like a 'home' visit can be stressful, and you might not look very confident or competent in the short time that is allowed for a home visit.

The home visit is an important part of the decision about where a person is going after a hospital stay. It is like an exam that you have to pass before they'll let you out. You only really get one go and you can't cram for it. The examiner has a high standard that they expect you to meet, because they've never lived with anyone as chaotic as you were before your admission. You've actually been this chaotic since your wife died twenty years ago and it's done you no harm, but they don't like it. You'll need to do better than that if you want them to say you'll be safe at home.

I told them I'd take my mom home now because the occupational therapist was on holiday and the home visit was postponed again for another few weeks. The nurse told me that if we discharged her without this OT [occupational therapist] test, social work would refuse to give her services. That would mean she'd get no home help. He was making it up as he went along but it spooked Mom into refusing to come home with me. (Son of Peterina, 86)

And sometimes the home visit turns out to be quite traumatic in itself:

Dad was bundled into the little van that the occupational therapists use and whisked off to his apartment, where they got him to try to make a cup of tea. He wasn't feeling very well and he had a different walking frame [walker] that he did not like, and in the course of it all he soiled himself. It's such a sad memory because he never went back to that apartment, and he'd had such happy times there. He'd not met the OT before. We were told he'd 'failed' his assessment. (Son of Jonathan, 87)

Getting out

We caught up with some shopping that day and went to a matinee at the pictures and grabbed some tea before we got to the hospital at visiting time, only to discover that she'd gone home in the ambulance while we were out and about … (Daughter of Alice, 79)

Sometimes your loved one will arrive home before you expected it. Don't be cross. Just be glad that they are home and prepare yourself for the fact that some of the community services might not have caught up with the hospital either. Sometimes when they are ready to come home, it takes a long time to get out of the system, which can seem worse.

Last time my mother left hospital, they got her dressed and sat at the end of the ward with her bag. Her bed was cleaned and someone else got in. Five hours she waited for her medication to be delivered from the hospital pharmacy. Five hours sitting in that chair, among all those sick people and their germs. Five hours. So this time she was coming out I took her home without the pills and went back and I sat waiting for the pills by myself. They weren't happy because they were supposed to explain them to her, but I told them I'd be doing that every ten minutes anyway, so they gave them to me and I left.

Don't get me wrong. They saved her life and I love them for that. They just don't have a clue about dementia. (Daughter of Aarika, 75)

chapter 13
Some legal, financial and ethical issues

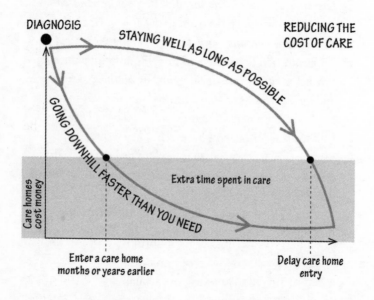

DIAGNOSIS

REDUCING THE COST OF CARE

STAYING WELL AS LONG AS POSSIBLE

GOING DOWNHILL FASTER THAN YOU NEED

Care homes cost money

Extra time spent in care

Enter a care home months or years earlier

Delay care home entry

If you have dementia you will probably reach a position where you won't be able to make decisions for yourself. There are robust legal processes that you can set up in advance to make sure that this does not lead to things happening to you outside the range of what you'd choose for yourself if you were on the case. You can set the controls while you are still able, and choose a person who will make proxy decisions for you if something completely unpredictable crops up. Because you know them and trust them and have spent time talking to them, you can relax and know that you'll be OK, since they know and understand what you want and can guess what you would have wanted if something unexpected happens. Getting wills and durable powers of attorney sorted is a smart move for any adult, but when you know you have dementia, you need to move quickly on these. At some later stage lawyers or doctors might have to stop listening to you because they realise you've reached the point where you lack the capacity to make a decision.

Those among you who need to know about these processes include people diagnosed or about to be diagnosed with dementia, their families and friends and those who work with them in care settings. Some of you may be asked to act as 'attorneys', 'agents' or 'guardians' and you might apply to be a 'receiver' or take on some other legal role. The law is really meant to be helpful, but it can't be helpful if you don't know how to use it and if you don't use it in time. The different mechanisms that are available and the differences between different countries and legal systems mean that technical terms you might encounter vary.

One obvious reason for attention to detail here is the real risk of financial and other forms of abuse of people with dementia because of their problem of lack of judgement. A recent study in the *New England Journal of Medicine* showed that this is the commonest form of elder abuse. Unfortunately, 90 per cent of perpetrators are family members, neighbours, friends or caregivers. Getting the legal position and financial systems sorted out protects family members against accusations of misusing anyone and protects the individual against abuse.

The AARP advises that you can safeguard the person's assets by closely monitoring their financial information on an ongoing basis. That way you could see if some rogue repair contractor has been billing them for non-existent work, or if amounts of cash have been withdrawn without any explanation. Theft should always be reported to law enforcement officers, but older people don't want to get relatives into trouble, and even if the perpetrator is a stranger, they are often too embarrassed to confess their own weakness. The AARP free newsletter includes information and scam alerts.

At the early stages of dementia you still have the capacity to do everything you ever did. As time goes by your capacity is judged by how well you understand and recall information and weigh up options. It might even be that you do understand but you are unable to demonstrate that you do, as sometimes happens with a stroke. That is why talking about all these matters well in advance is really important. At your fiftieth birthday party, when you are in your prime, is not too soon.

If the person with dementia can no longer make their own decisions, they are not legally able to assign a power of attorney. In law, you need to fully understand what is going on if you are signing away legal responsibilities. Some powers of attorney work at once, and stop when you lose capacity to decide – so they are not very useful for situations of cognitive impairment like dementia – and others don't actually come into force until the day you are unable to make a decision.

I'm in my fifties with no sign of a stroke or dementia or anything and no one in my family had any of that so I'm not worried. But I have had a number of conversations with my daughter over the years, right from when she was quite young. She'd sometimes say, 'That's enough …' and walk away, apparently bored, but in fact I've discovered she was retaining it all. Now she has hit the legal age, we've got the power of attorney sorted so, if or when something happens to me, she can take over. I've told her that if I'm in a home and don't know her any more she doesn't need to be sad, but just check them out regularly to make sure they are doing the right thing. I know and love her now enough for all my life and the life to come. What might happen after dementia does not matter to me. (Fatma, 56)

A person who no longer has the capacity to understand a complex issue like managing a portfolio of shares or selling a house might still be capable of deciding what to wear, what to eat and where to go on holiday. So capacity is not an 'all or nothing' issue.

Advance decisions

There are different names for the process of making a statement about how you'd like to be treated in future when and if you lose the capacity to express an opinion. They are called 'living wills', 'advance statements', 'advance directives' or 'advance decisions'. In some cases there is a technical difference between these, but you will find people using them interchangeably. When you are ill and can't speak for yourself, such as after an accident, doctors and nurses have a legal obligation to act in your best interests and often they decide that for themselves, particularly in an emergency, and ask questions later.

Advance statements tell others that you have decided in advance that you want them not to put you through a particular process or procedure or treatment. An example is a statement by a Jehovah's Witness that he or she must not be given a blood transfusion, even if the doctor believes it will save that person's life. Who knows about the existence of your statement and where it is stored is clearly very important. Some women might have it in their handbag or purse but maybe no one will look there in time. Some people have their advance statement in a safety deposit box, which is not very accessible. It is useful if crucial people, including your doctor, know about and record your wishes. This is why living will registries have been set up in the United States and other countries. Documents are on file so that the family or health care provider can check what the patient wanted, even when the patient is no longer able to speak for themselves. A living will can be changed and updated, and at the time it is needed, how much weight is placed on it will depend to an extent on how long ago it was made.

What might you be thinking about?

Your advance decision might be to refuse treatment, even if that causes your death. You can't insist on treatment, only refuse treatment. In the UK, doctors are legally bound by your advance decision in England and Wales, and in Scotland and Northern Ireland their insurers advise them that it's regulated by common law and that the courts are likely to support a clear directive from the patient. So even in one small country like the UK, there are different positions. So whatever country you live in, it is a good idea to discuss advance decisions with your doctor and make sure it is in your notes to have the best chance of control over what happens next, if you lose capacity. Tell the family too, in case the medics do not see this message in your notes in time and just ask the family for an opinion in the meantime. The last thing you want is for everyone to have done their best – only to say 'Oops' the next day when they discover your note, while you are vegetating in intensive care after an aggressive and perhaps relatively unsuccessful attempt to resuscitate you.

In some places if you are trying to say in advance that you want to refuse 'life-sustaining' treatment like artificial nutrition or hydration even if your life is at risk, the decision has to be in writing and signed by you and witnessed. An example might be that you decide, if you have dementia and subsequently develop cancer, you don't want it to be treated but want to be kept comfortable and die naturally. (Interestingly, research shows that people with dementia get less cancer than the general population.) A more likely scenario is that a person with dementia might get pneumonia or suffer a stroke. Pneumonia used to be called 'the old man's friend'. People died of it peacefully in their sleep. Now that we can treat it intensively with antibiotics and intravenous infusions and life support, you are less likely to die from it. But you could choose in advance to say you don't want those treatments. It's important to know that you can't use an advance decision to demand assisted suicide or euthanasia if it is not legal in your country but you can ask for nature to be allowed to take its course while you are given tender loving care. In any case you should review it regularly and you can cancel it at any time.

In the Netherlands advance directives requesting euthanasia are legally recognised but research on what happens in the Netherlands indicates that advance directives for euthanasia are not normally adhered to in the case of older people with advanced dementia. The majority of people with dementia are admitted to a nursing home and die there and their treatment there might be limited, particularly if the euthanasia request is known about. Some people with dementia in the early stage have asked for and received euthanasia, but it is interesting that the opinions of relatives and care home residents do not always match. Humans constantly adapt to the situation in which they find themselves and what we might think in advance would be unbearable, may not turn out to be so. The difficult thing is that when euthanasia is used for dementia, it has to be carried out when the patient is still competent. It is therefore given in advance of the condition that the patient decides will be intolerable. In fact, the patient can't know this. It is a disturbing thought.

You might decide that if the time for hard choices comes you want someone else to make that decision at that time about the sorts of issues that would otherwise be captured in your advance statement. You do this by making that person your attorney. You do this by creating a power of attorney, or lasting power of attorney or enduring power of attorney. Again, the attorney takes your views into account but they are not legally bound by them. In many legal systems there are two sorts of attorney. One is for property and financial affairs, the other for health decisions. The second is sometimes called a 'health care proxy'. It's this person in particular who needs to know about any advance decision about life-sustaining treatment, as they will be in a position if there is any debate about what to do, to tell the medical staff on your behalf.

So an advance statement can be:

◆ an advance decision that refuses specific treatments, like resuscitation from a heart attack;

◆ a more generalised statement that says 'no life-sustaining treatments if I've got no chance of getting better';

◆ a plea to 'give me everything that is available at the time';

◆ a statement of values, not just about clinical care and treatment but about what life means to you – for example, 'life in a dependent state when I don't know my relatives is of no value to me';

◆ a statement of who should be consulted (if this is a person to whom you've given welfare power of attorney they can actually make decisions, not just be consulted).

What is mental capacity?

The guiding principle is that a person has the right to be assumed to have capacity to make their own decisions unless someone proves otherwise, but dementia forces people into ethical and practical grey areas. All practicable steps have to be taken to support the person with dementia in making decisions for themselves. And they must be allowed to make eccentric or unwise decisions. One problem is that not all doctors are well equipped to assess capacity.

If you ask my mum anything in the afternoon she always says, 'NO!' and I'm pretty sure she has no idea what is being suggested. Yet, the next morning, and every morning, she'll enter into a sensible conversation about the same thing. (Eleanor, talking about her mother, Jane, 80)

Dementia is overwhelmingly tiring, and if you check out the person in a darkened room late on in the day when they are hungry and thirsty and just waking from a nap, they won't make as much sense as they could at another time of the day. Is this not true of all of us to an extent? It's just that the rest of us are not at risk of someone overriding our decisions because they think we're not very smart. You will know when the best time of day is to give the person the best chance of thinking about what they really want.

Another principle is that if a decision is made on my behalf the person making it needs to prove that they're doing so in my best interest, and that the least restrictive decision is being made. So you might think that I can't manage my finances, but I can still have enough money for shopping for shoes you think are expensive and unsuitable. The vexed question is sometimes about who decides:

The lawyer would not let George change his will because he wasn't sure if he had the mental capacity, and she said we needed to ask the doctor. The doctor said that wasn't a clinical decision – it was a legal one. George was stuck in the middle. (Wife, 71)

Practical suggestions about money

Investment News in the United States has reported that financial advisers are discarding clients if the firm can't be sure where the liability lies when confusing and difficult scenarios arise, as when a person with dementia is probably being scammed by someone.

But reaching out – even to family members – risks being in violation of privacy laws.

While at least one state, Washington, has passed legislation that affords advisers more leniency in making referrals or refusing to execute a suspicious transaction,

*there are no universal guidelines, said Andrea Seidt,
the Ohio securities commissioner and president of the
National Association of State Securities Administrators.
(www.investmentnews.com/article/20141103/
FEATURE/141039973/unraveling-minds)*

All of us need to be prepared as early as possible. Apart from making a power of attorney, there are steps that you can take to make life simple for yourself and your family.

For years my mother kept telling me every time I visited where she kept their financial records. She died before Dad and he never had understood their finances, even while she was alive. She made sure that we knew where all the documents were, and where the keys and codes where. It was all in a big folder in a drawer, along with details of their monthly expenses. Dad worried about his income after she passed away but because we had all the information we were able to reassure him and to take over those affairs quite smoothly. She was so clever and I'm going to do that for my daughter, well in advance. (Jane, 59)

If a bank becomes aware that an account holder has lost mental capacity, it will freeze the account until an attorney or a court order intervenes. While you still have capacity, setting up some of the following mechanisms might make life easier later:

◆ Arrange as many automated payments and standing orders as you can so that bills get paid regularly without you having to handle them.

◆ Think about having a special small joint bank account with the person who has power of attorney. This means that he or she can access any of your money that is in that account, and if you trust each other, that is convenient. While you are unwell or in hospital you could say, 'Send a cheque from our joint account to Doris for her birthday,' and it would be done. Or you could say, 'When you are in town, will you get me out some cash from the ATM?' and they can just do that and bring it to you.

◆ Think about a third-party mandate. This is an instruction to your bank or building society to provide access to your account for another person. However, if you lose capacity, the mandate is terminated, so it's not that useful for dementia in the later stages.

How to pay for dementia care?

Dementia costs many countries billions of dollars every year, making it among the biggest drains on their health and social care systems. Analysis has been made of the social care costs – such as care provided by family members and in those countries where they have them, live in maids or foreign domestic workers. The price tag is expected to grow exponentially as the world population ages.

Family income is lost when caregivers take time off work, and dementia incurs direct healthcare costs, including hospital admissions and doctor visits. Professional care, such as rehabilitation services, or care for a patient's daily needs, is almost never free at the point of delivery. Supported housing, day centres and ultimately residential care are often surprisingly expensive.

All over the world, the majority of care is still provided by families. The individual requirement for personal and family contribution is actually increasing in countries that have previously had government subsidies for care. Calls for more government support intensify as families discover the cost of caring for increasing numbers of older relatives, but even where there is a government goal of universal access, there is a realisation that this is not affordable or sustainable for most administrations. A multi-layered financing system is more common with contributions from personal savings, family time or cash, insurance products, charity and government or local authority funding.

It is impossible in a book such as this to describe the financing arrangements in each country because the situation is complex and constantly changing within and between institutions. Even if your health and social care provider gives you some information about financial support, it is necessary to do further homework on how to pay, or to discover how to get support for paying.

A number of countries have taken the first step of formulating strategies and plans. You can find details for your own country on www.alz.co.uk which is the website for Alzheimer's Disease International. Here you will also find up to date links to the Alzheimer organisation in your own country. This is a good starting point for information about funding.

In addition to Alzheimer or dementia specific charities you may discover that other charities can help at this time, for example, special funds for Veterans, or funds from your church or faith group. Financial institutions are starting to take heed of the need for savings and insurance plans which can be considered earlier in life, either for personal or parental care.

Contacts for some national Alzheimer organisations

Australia
Alzheimer's Australia
Tel: +61 2 6278 8900
Helpline: 1800 100 500
Email support: helpline.nat@alzheimers.org.au
Email national office: nat.admin@alzheimers.org.au
Web: fightdementia.org.au

Bermuda
Alzheimer's Family Support Group
Tel: +441 238 2168 (pm)
Email: JulieKay@ibl.bm

Canada
Alzheimer Society of Canada
Tel: +1 416 488 8772
Helpline: 1800 616 8816
Fax: +1 416 488 3778
Email: info@alzheimer.ca
Web: www.alzheimer.ca

Cyprus
Pancyprian Association of Alzheimer's Disease
Tel: +357 24 627 104
Fax: +357 24 627 106
Email: alzhcyprus@cytanet.com.cy

Gibraltar
The Gibraltar Alzheimer's and Dementia Society
Tel: +350 2007 1049
Email: gads@gibtelecom.net

Hong Kong SAR
Hong Kong Alzheimer's Disease Association
Tel: +852 23 381 120
Carer Hotline: +852 23 382 277
Fax: +852 23 38 0772
Email: headoffice@hkada.org.hk
Web: www.hkada.org.hk

India
Alzheimer's and Related Disorders Society of India
Tel: +91 4885 223 801
Email: ardsinationaloffice@gmail.com
Web: www.ardsi.org

Ireland
Alzheimer Society of Ireland
Tel: +353 1 284 6616
Helpline: +353 1 800 341 341
Fax: +353 1 284 6030
Email: info@alzheimer.ie
Web: www.alzheimer.ie

Kenya
Alzheimer's & Dementia Organisation
Tel: +254 723471096
Email: info@alzkenya.org
Web: http://alzkenya.org

Malta
Malta Dementia Society
Email: info@maltadementiasociety.org.mt
Web: www.maltadementiasociety.org.mt

New Zealand
Alzheimers New Zealand
Tel: +64 4 387 8264
Helpline: 0800 004 001
Fax: +64 4 387 9682
Email: admin@alzheimers.org.nz
Web: www.alzheimers.org.nz

Pakistan
Alzheimer's Pakistan
Tel: +92 42 759 6589
Fax: +92 42 757 3911
Email: info@alz.org.pk
Web: www.alz.org.pk

Philippines
Alzheimer's Disease Association of the Philippines
Tel/fax: +632 723 1039
Email: info@alzphilippines.com
Web: www.alzphilippines.com

Singapore
Alzheimer's Disease Association
Tel: +65 6353 8734
Fax: +65 6353 8518
Email: adahq@alz.org.sg
Web: www.alz.org.sg

South Africa
Alzheimer's South Africa
Tel: +27 11 792 2511/8387
Fax: +27 11 792 7135
Helpline: 0860 102 681 (Mornings from 09h00)
Email: info@alzheimers.org.za
Web: www.alzheimers.org.za

Trinidad and Tobago
Alzheimer's Association of Trinidad and Tobago
Tel: +1 868 622 6134 or +1 868 632 1168
Email: nebinniss@gmail.com or alztrinbago@gmail.com

It is a good idea to get some practical advice about organising finances, asking some key questions: Has someone been named to look after financial interests? Are financial and legal documents, such as wills, insurance policies and bank accounts gathered together in a safe location? And have financial priorities been set?

In addition to the above, gather the following legal and financial documents and information, and let a trusted adviser and family member know where they are stored:

◆ Bank accounts
◆ Credit cards
◆ Loans and mortgages
◆ Insurance policies (life, auto, home, disability)
◆ Pension plans and RRSPs
◆ Investments
◆ Real estate, home, business, car ownership
◆ Prepaid funeral arrangements and/or cemetery plot

The final ethical issue

Unfortunately, at the time of writing, there is no cure for dementia. My friends with dementia have, however, taught me that being diagnosed early is a great benefit, because it lets you know that the time has come to get on with your bucket list, while you can, and to tell everyone you love that you do in fact love them, and remind them where you've left things, and take time to have fun while there is still time for fun.

Everyone involved with dementia has good reason to be sad, because it comes at the end of life, and that's when we all go our separate ways. I hope that knowledge of how to help with the difficult parts of this path will make it easier for people to help each other along the way, or for those of us with dementia to travel it ourselves.

Peace, my heart, let the time for the parting be sweet.
Let it not be a death but completeness.

Let love melt into memory and pain into songs.
Let the flight through the sky end in the folding of the wings over the nest.
Let the last touch of your hands be gentle like the flower of the night.
Stand still, O Beautiful End, for a moment, and say your last words in silence.
I bow to you and hold up my lamp to light you on your way.

Rabindranath Tagore

chapter 14

Afterword: dementia is a feminist issue

In 2015, when I was at the Dementia Services Development Centre at the University of Stirling, with the support of the Dementia Services Development Trust, I conducted a survey to determine how thinking about dementia had changed over the previous twenty-five years. We had seen media reports that people today are more afraid of dementia than cancer, and we wanted to know if that was true. Did people believe, as has been reported, that health and social care workers do not provide care based on research evidence? What plans did people think they needed to make for their loved one? Nearly 3,000 people completed the survey. Although we tried very hard to get both men and women to complete the survey, men were much less likely to do so. The most remarkable finding was that the men who did complete the survey differed radically from the women in how they think about dementia:

◆ Although most people know that dementia is caused by an underlying disease, men are twice as likely as women to regard dementia as part of normal aging.

◆ Men are also more likely than women to believe that people with dementia can be cured.

◆ More men than women believe that drugs are or will be the answer.

◆ Men seem to have greater confidence than women that how patients with dementia are treated in hospitals is based on research.

◆ More men than women believe that you and your family should contribute to care, either by providing it or by paying for it.

◆ When asked, men had more confidence than women that better awareness in the community would help with dementia, but women had a stronger belief that improving the knowledge of care staff is needed.

◆ Women are much more aware of the dangers of a hospital admission than men are.

◆ More women than men have a negative experience of being listened to by the health care system.

◆ More women than men fear dementia and say they'd rather die than be affected by it.

◆ More women than men responded positively to the idea of voluntary euthanasia.

Looking at these raw data, we wondered whether this difference between genders was a modern phenomenon. And how much had the way people regard dementia changed, even in our own professional lifetimes and in the history of the Dementia Services Development Trust?

In the 1970s, just before the Dementia Centre was created, institutional care for people with dementia was improving but still included some dreadful practices.

Health care workers performed their tasks as fast as possible so that they could sit down for a cup of tea and a cigarette. To speed up the bathing routine, for example, patients would be stripped naked in front of each other in a production line.

When I was a nursing student in a large psychiatric hospital in the 1980s, more enlightened textbooks suggested that curtains be hung between the bathtubs in the bathroom so that patients could not see each other but the nurse could still supervise them all. I saw people tied to the toilet pan so that they wouldn't leave the bathroom while staff fetched other patients. Even in those days, any staff or students who complained about this sort of humiliation would be labelled as squeamish and unsuitable for nursing work with people who had dementia. A good nurse was someone who could 'bathe and toilet' a lot of people quickly. That task was made easier by heaps of communal apparel, which allowed nursing staff to dress people in whatever was at hand, including dresses for women with slit openings at the back to make it easier for staff to manhandle them in the toilet. People who could still walk were put in wheelchairs and hurled along corridors because they did not move fast enough for the staff. Eventually they would lose the power to walk unaided purely because they were not allowed to take time to continue doing things for themselves. The situation is much better now, but the horror of institutional care in former times still taints how we think about dementia today.

Surveys make most sense if you compare them with a baseline, and unfortunately, there is no proper baseline for how people in general used to think about dementia. We know that people twenty to thirty years ago did not speak much about dementia, and a lot of what was said was wrong. In addition, because a lot of what has been written in the past was written by men, it is hard to make a gendered analysis of what people were thinking.

It is said that before the rise of the Victorian institutions, 'the family' used to take care of old people. What caused this norm to change from home care to institutional care? I believe that because family care is usually done by women, the increased opportunities for women in the workplace may have been a key factor in the creation of institutions. Is it more cost effective for your daughter to stay at home and look after you or for her to go out to work? Which of these two options can the family best afford? As more women entered the workplace and obtained higher-paying jobs, and as family size decreased, institutions came into their own.

Today, however, most people with dementia are living in their own homes, even if they have no family. As the cost of care homes rises, will women again in future forgo opportunities to work or study because they need to care for their frail older parents? And how does all this affect the way people think about dementia?

The preponderance of women looking after people with dementia suggests that women have a greater reason to take an interest in old age, frailty and dementia than men. In our own dementia centre, male employees – including academics, managers and others

– had never been more than 10 per cent of the staff. Later we began to examine the gender balance of the people who create government policies on dementia.

A global research review had already been undertaken by Alzheimer's Disease International in 2015. The purpose of that report was to understand the dementia-related issues affecting women internationally. The report looked at women living with dementia, women caring for people with dementia in a professional role, and women undertaking an informal caregiving role for someone with dementia. The report also looked at factors affecting women in low- and middle-income countries, at family structures and kinship, and at the effect of migration on women.

The key findings of this report are startling. The prevalence of dementia is higher in women, and they live with more severe symptoms. They are more likely to be informal carers or even professional carers. The report noted that there is very little research on the gender issues in dementia.

Over 60 per cent of people with dementia are female. This is partly because women live longer and dementia is related to age. But that is not all. As this book has explained, dementia is not a disease but the symptom of any of a range of diseases, the commonest of which is Alzheimer's. In contrast to other diseases, the severity of the symptoms is not always directly related to the severity of the underlying disease. Symptoms are made worse by depression, loneliness, poor diet and lack of exercise – problems that are worse for anyone who has fewer resources.

The current generation of older women – particularly married women – have often depended on a man's occupational pension in old age because these women had mainly worked at home performing domestic and caregiving tasks. Until relatively recent times, if a man and a woman divorced, the woman's unwaged contribution to the family resources would probably not be compensated, leaving her in poverty in old age even if her husband was still alive. Even today, the death of a husband or partner can leave a woman who has never participated in the workforce in difficult financial circumstances. The same is true for a man who loses his partner, but he is more likely to have earned and saved more and is more likely to have benefited from an occupational pension. So in general, older women are likely to be less well off than men, and being poor makes some of the things that would reduce dementia symptoms simply unaffordable.

Research shows that stress in midlife is related to dementia in later life, and in many cases women's lives in the last century have been more stressful than men's because of lower pay and less financial security in old age, less protection against sex discrimination and violence, and the hazards of childbirth, among other things. Research also shows other ways in which women can be disproportionately affected by dementia and old age frailty.

Workers in dementia care, who are mainly women, earn low wages and are often not held in high esteem, which is reflected in their working conditions.

When an older woman has a husband with dementia

she often has the life skills to care for him, so he is more likely to end his days in reasonable comfort at home, especially as she is probably a little bit younger than he is. When an older woman has dementia, the reverse is often true – her husband may not have the skills to care for her, so she is more likely to end her days not in comfort and not at home, especially since he is probably a bit older than she is – which is another reason why a disproportionate number of residents in care homes are women.

Men may be caregivers for their elderly parents, but most of this work falls on daughters, granddaughters, and nieces.

Midlife stress raises the likelihood of dementia in women, and older women have often experienced stresses that we will never know. How recently did unmarried women have their children ripped away from them for adoption or deportation in an atmosphere of violence and disgrace? What other painful and stressful secrets might they carry related to previous miscarriages or abortions that could not be discussed?

These statements should not be misinterpreted as a diatribe from someone who does not like men and refuses to recognise their contribution, which is often as heroic as any women's. But the statistics do not lie. We need to celebrate the lives of the older women we care for now that they are in their eighties and nineties. These women were the pioneers who did without many of the benefits that they subsequently won for us – such as maternity leave and allowances, equal rights at work, laws that work against violence and rape, recognition of the need for education for girls, decent sanitary products, washing machines and disposable nappies.

The difference in how men and women regard euthanasia needs to be explored more carefully. It is not clear whether those who would rather die are afraid of being humiliated and badly cared for or whether they would prefer to avoid the cost of that care so that they can leave a legacy for their children. It appears that men may have more confidence that science will find a cure for dementia, and that is not in itself a bad thing unless it distracts us from the need to provide care and support now, to the women (and men) who are most affected by this sometimes cruel affliction.

Although bad things still happen in a care setting, the situation in general is much better now than it was in the early 1980s. The ideal of support at home followed if needed by a move to a homelike setting is a reality for many people. Good meals, exercise, entertainment, company, privacy, dignity – all of these are expected now. But I wanted to know whether that has made a difference in how people think about dementia. It is always frustrating that every research report ends by saying, 'More research is needed.' But in this case it is all too true.

Those people and organisations that are shaping policy about dementia need to defend themselves against a possible accusation that men are making policy decisions about what is essentially a women's issue. A quick glance at the executives of a number of elected bodies, advocacy organisations and research establishments reflects the current prevalence of men at the top in business and society. This must change in all walks of life, but change in organisations that are shaping policy about dementia is urgent in light of what we are learning about the difference in attitudes towards dementia between men and women. The voices of women caregivers and women with dementia must be heard and must have a role in shaping policy.

Helpful organisations

Alzheimer's Disease International www.alz.co.uk 'believes that the key to winning the fight against dementia lies in a unique association of Global Solutions and local knowledge. As such, it works locally, by empowering national Alzheimer associations to promote and offer care and support for people with dementia and their carers, whilst working globally to focus attention on the epidemic and campaign for policy change from governments and the World Health Organization.'

Alzheimer Europe www.alzheimer-europe.org is an organisation representing 36 European Alzheimer associations. It is a non-governmental organisation aimed at raising awareness of all forms of dementia by creating a common European platform through co-ordination and co-operation between Alzheimer organisations throughout Europe. Alzheimer Europe is also a source of information on all aspects of dementia.

In the USA the **Alzheimer's Association** www.alz.org works on a global, national and local level to enhance care and support for all those affected by Alzheimer's and other dementias. They have local chapters across the USA. Their free online tool, Alzheimer's Navigator www.alzheimersnavigator.org provides individuals with Alzheimer's and their caregivers with step-by-step guidance and customised action plans, and their website is packed with information that can help caregivers, professionals and people with dementia.

Alzheimer's Australia www.fightdementia.org.au provides a national dementia helpline for people with dementia, their caregivers, families and friends, health professionals, service providers, community organisations, students and people seeking information. They also provide Help Sheets on useful topics, counselling, and family carer education in addition to public awareness activities.

The Alzheimer Society of Bangladesh www.alzheimerbd.com is a non-government, non-profit, voluntary organisation based in Dhaka. It was established by a group of social workers, caregivers and doctors in 2006 to improve quality of life. It carries out a wide range of programmes, for example, awareness raising, education, training and research, rendering support to people with dementia and caregivers.

The Alzheimer Society of Canada www.alzheimer.ca is the nationwide health charity for people living with Alzheimer's disease and other dementias. Active in communities right across Canada, the Society partners with Alzheimer Societies in every Canadian province to offer information, support and education programmes for people with dementia, their families and caregivers. ASC funds research to find a cure and improve the care of people with dementia, promotes public education and awareness of Alzheimer's disease and other dementias, and influences policy and decision-making to address the needs of people with dementia and their caregivers.

The Hong Kong Alzheimer's Disease Association www.hkada.org.hk/ provides specialised services to people with dementia. Running on a fully self-financed, non-profit making basis, without Government subsidy, it aims to provide professional and multi-therapeutic activities and services to people with dementia and their caregivers. It also provides different levels of training and education to professionals, caregivers and the public, to enhance their knowledge and skills to achieve the effects of 'Early Detection, Early Treatment, Early Planning'.

The Alzheimer's and Related Disorders Society of India www.ardsi.org/ founded by Dr Jacob Roy has spread its activities across India. At present ARDSI has Chapters in New Delhi, Pune, Manipur, Jaipur, Lucknow, Mumbai, Greater Mumbai, Kolkata, Hyderabad, Chennai, Bangalore, Goa, Coimbatore, Calicut, Cochin, Kottayam, Pathanamthitta and Trivandrum, along with support groups attached to the Chapters.

The Alzheimer Society of Ireland www.alzheimer.ie/ works across the country in local communities providing dementia specific services and support and advocating for the rights and needs of people living with dementia and their carers. A non-profit organisation, it operates the Alzheimer National Helpline offering information and support to anyone affected by dementia.

Alzheimer's Disease Foundation (Malaysia)

www.adfm.org.my/ Aims to generate awareness and support for dementia. It offers a list of support groups or contacts in the different states of Malaysia with meetings and activities organised for each locality. It provides medical and other references of interest to those seeking specialist advice/ treatment, information on Alzheimer's disease. Stories and articles selected from their Support Group newsletter 'Sharing' enable Alzheimer's families to keep up to date with the big Malaysian Alzheimer's family. There is a calendar of events, and opportunities to participate.

The Malta Dementia Society

www.maltadementiasociety.org.mt/ is a non-governmental and non-profit organisation for persons with dementia, their carers, families and friends. The society brings together healthcare professionals and interested persons to increase the knowledge of dementia and its care. They provide leaflets, publications and newsletters.

Alzheimer's New Zealand www.alzheimers.org.nz/ represents people affected by dementia at a national level by raising awareness of dementia, providing information and resources for people affected by dementia, advocating for high quality services for people affected by dementia, and promoting research about prevention, treatment, cure and care of people affected by dementia. It supports a federation of 21 local Alzheimer's NZ organisations throughout New Zealand, each of which provides a range of supports.

Alzheimer's Pakistan www.alz.org.pk/ is registered with Punjab Social Welfare Department and the objective of this non-government community organisation is the welfare of people with dementia and their care givers. Since 1999, it has been in the forefront to create mass awareness about dementias and actively involved in developing services like day care, memory clinic, support group and training programmes for family members, doctors and social workers. Run by volunteers from all walks of life.

Alzheimer's Disease Association, Singapore http://www.alz.org.sg/ was formed in 1990 as a result of growing concern for the needs of people with dementia and their families. ADA is a voluntary welfare organisation and is made up of caregivers, professionals and all who are interested in dementia. It provides a wide range of services including day care, transportation, information, training, counseling for caregivers and other services in English, Mandarin and Malay.

Alzheimers South Africa http://www.alzheimers.org.za/ has a range of local services and activities including support groups which can be located via their regional offices across South Africa.

Alzheimer Iberoamerica-AIB

http://alzheimeriberoamerica.org/ es una Federación Internacional de Asociaciones y Fundaciones de Alzheimer, integrada por miembros plenos en 21 países iberoamericanos.

An international federation of Alzheimer's associations and foundations comprising full members in twenty-one Latin American countries.

Resources

Key Dementia Services Development Centre resources

The following are available from Amazon or from the Dementia Shop: http://www.dementiashop.co.uk/

◆ June Andrews and Allan House, *10 Helpful Hints for Carers: Practical Solutions for Carers Living with People with Dementia*. This is an easy-to-read guide for carers living with people with dementia. It provides simple, practical solutions to the everyday problems family caregivers can face when looking after a person with dementia. Covering areas like how to cope with aggression, creating relaxing environments, 'wandering' and sleeplessness and how to cope with dementia and depression, it is a mine of information and good advice.

◆ Dementia Services Development Centre, *10 Helpful Hints for Dementia Design at Home: Practical Design Solutions for Carers Living at Home with Someone Who Has Dementia*. This is an easy-to-read guide for caregivers of people with dementia. It provides simple and practical design solutions to adapt the living environment for people with dementia so that they can live independently for as long as possible. Covering topics such as lighting, interior décor, sound and the use of assistive technology it gives advice on how these elements can be used to their best advantage in the homes of people with dementia.

◆ June Andrews, *10 Helpful Hints for when a Person with Dementia Has to Go to Hospital*. People with dementia can't avoid going to hospital, even though it can be hazardous for them. Based on *Dementia: The One-Stop Guide* by Professor June Andrews, this book gives practical hints for families and friends on how you can help a patient with dementia survive a hospital admission.

Children's books about dementia

◆ Sarah Lynn, *Tip-Tap Pop*: Rosa finds a way to communicate through dancing.

◆ Maria Shriver, *What's Happening to Grandpa*: Kate explores ways of helping herself and her grandfather by creating a photo album of memories.

◆ Linda Jacobs Altman, *Singing with Momma Lou*: nine-year-old Tamika dreads visiting her grandmother in the nursing home, but overcomes this with help from her father.

◆ Irene Mackay, *The Forgetful Elephant*: a story of how a little elephant copes when her grandfather starts to forget her.

Acknowledgements

I want to thank Andrew Franklin, Penny Daniel and the staff of Profile Books for encouragement and advice in putting this book together.

My own knowledge is enriched by many conversations with people who live with dementia, in particular Dr James McKillop, and I thank Dr Cesar Rodriguez at the Dementia Services Development Trust, and the Trustees for their professional advice and financial support. All those have worked and volunteered at the Dementia Services Development Centre at the University of Stirling have shaped my thinking on these matters and supported the development of these ideas.

Thanks are due to my husband Charles and daughter Charlotte who give me support to write. I am also thankful for the support of colleagues, members of my family and friends, including Mark Butler, Professor Allan House, Sarah Lenz Lock, Sonia Mangan, Maureen McGinn, Nigel Robb, Professor Kenneth Rockwood and Mary Schulz who read drafts and put up with my absence while I was writing.

Index